Bischko

An Introduction to Acupuncture

An Introduction to Acupuncture

By Prof. Johannes Bischko MD

Translated by Diana Reese-Soltész

2nd Revised and Expanded Edition

With 22 Figures

HAUG

Karl F Haug Publishers, Heidelberg

Short title:

Bischko, Johannes:
An introduction to acupuncture / by Johannes Bischko. Transl. by Diana Reese-Soltész. – 2nd rev. and expanded ed. – Heidelberg: Haug, 1985.
Einheitssacht.: Einführung in die Akupunktur «engl.»
ISBN 3-7760-0842-3

2nd revised and expanded edition 1985

Publisher's number: 8542
ISBN: 3-7760-0842-3
Layout by Karl F. Haug Verlag GmbH & Co

Typeset and printed by Heinrich Schreck KG, Maikammer, Federal Republic of Germany

CONTENTS

FOREWORD

My English-speaking colleagues who maintain contact with our institute or were trained here encouraged me to publish this book in English. In the last seven years, the original German-language version has become the most widely-read acupuncture book in German-speaking countries and is now in its 10th edition.

The Viennese Acupuncture School represents a combination of traditional, and particularly, modern medical concepts based on recent research. Perhaps it is just this mixture which appeals to the reader. I hope that this book will reach as wide an audience in English-speaking countries as it has here in Europe. The style and structure of the book is adapted to the needs of the medical practitioner. It should serve not only as a textbook for the beginning acupuncturist, but also as a source of reference for those physicians who already have had more experience with the method.

Today, sufficient data exists which has succeeded in bringing acupuncture out of the realm of mysticism and quackery. Furthermore, acupuncture has given new impetus to many other fields of research. Therefore, today we can say with certainty that every physician should have at least some basic knowledge of acupuncture, and this book will certainly be of aid.

There are many people whom I would like to thank for encouraging me to have my book translated. These are my American colleagues, and especially Diana REESE-SOLTÉSZ, who translated my book in the most conscientious manner possible. This was no easy task indeed, especially as many German terms and expressions often sound the same as they do in English, but have a completely different meaning. She took her work very seriously, gave the rough drafts to several physicians (Drs. GENCHEFF, OLMS, PONTASCH, RILEY, SCHAEFER, and E. BRAUNEIS, L. A. C. S. T., to whom I would like to express my gratitude) for review, and gratefully followed their advice.

I would also like to express my thanks again to my colleagues, FEUCHT, KROPEJ, KRÖTLINGER, MENG, PETRICEK, and ZEITLER for their suggestions regarding the original German-language version, as well as to my wife who has given me much understanding and valuable criticism.

Vienna, May, 1978

Johannes J. BISCHKO, M. D.
Head of the Ludwig
Boltzmann Acupuncture
Institute, Vienna

Johannes Bischko, An Introduction to Acupuncture

Note:

Some authors refer to acupuncture meridians (Kings) as channels.

Acupuncture points are sometimes referred to as loci.

Bladder: B is sometimes referred to as Bl.

Kidney: K is sometimes referred to as Ki.

Triple Heater: 3 H is sometimes referred to as TrH or Triple Warmer: TrW.

Gallbladder: G is sometimes referred to as GB.

Pilot Vessel: PV is sometimes referred to as Governor Vessel: GV.

FOREWORD TO THE SECOND, REVISED AND EXPANDED EDITION

A second edition of "the Introduction" having been called for is not only gratifying, but also provided a welcome opportunity to bring the text up to date, iron out some discrepancies present in the first edition, and expand in a number of areas in keeping with the 13th German-language edition, as well as the newest research results. Hence, you will find in this edition, among others, a new chapter devoted entirely to research, an appendix containing an overview of the meridians, as well as the Chinese names of the points now being given in Pinyin in place of the French transcription used hithertofore. And so, I also have the pleasant task of heartily thanking my collabrorators, Dr. *Liertzer,* for compilation of the overview, which will facilitate comprehension of the network of acupuncture, its meridians and points, and Dr. *Meng,* for the drawings and his help regarding the Chinese nomenclature. My appreciation also goes to Dr. *Heinzl* for his constructive suggestions. And special thanks to the translator, *Diana Reese-Soltész,* who painstakingly scrutinized, revised, and expanded the text.

It is my hope that my readers will also comprehend this edition as an expression of my honest efforts and desire to create a Western method of acupuncture and to promote the use thereof.

Vienna, July, 1985

Prof. *Johannes Bischko, M.D.*

INTRODUCTION

"So many new things may be learned from the past."

Our times have brought with them an abundance of newly-acquired knowledge of natural science and seemingly unlimited technological possibilities, these offering increasingly exact diagnostic aids. They have led to turbulent developments in medicine, which – difficult to grasp in their entirety – have necessitated ever more splitter groups of ever more specialized or partial disciplines. Despite all this, a way of seeing man and body as a whole is still indispensable – but it has been forced into the background in the process.

Interest in old, forgotten methods has once again increased, especially on account of the rising number of functional diseases. This even more so as it is just these disorders which can be grasped only with difficulty using common diagnostics – based on the prevailing cellular pathological laws – and which, in many cases, also prove to be accessible to conventional therapeutic measures only with difficulty if at all.

Recall also the various injurious side effects of many drugs, or allergies thereto, and that, for whatever reasons, many diseases have changed in the course of time, today presenting themselves in different – usually shortened or masked – forms.

This is where classical acupuncture, adopted from ancient China, gives us today an answer, which does not seem evident at first glance. Classical acupuncture always tries to take a causal approach to a disease, as a rule in a way which we in modern times may distinguish as reinstatement of vegetative regulation or of vegetative equilibrium.

It will therefore prove to be especially effective whenever common therapeutic measures have brought unsatisfactory results. This is unfortunately the case to an ever-increasing degree nowadays. Recall not only allergies to certain drugs, but, even more so, the contra-indications thereof because of possible damaging side effects. In contrast, properly executed, acupuncture will never cause injury or injurious side effects.

Through its language and comparisons, it is this book's aim to show points in common with conventional medicine, and to bridge differences. Hence, in keeping with literature on acupuncture, it is written in a rather unorthodox manner, therewith, however, facilitating a conventionally-trained physician's confrontation with the material. This results not in small part from my own experiences therewith. Because in the past, left on one's own, it was very hard to work out the essentials from the myriad of traditional hand-me-down data. I have therefore intentionally deleted all philosophy, which, though very interesting, tends to scare off the novice. A number of other ways of approaching the material have also been left out on purpose.

I wish to close this brief introduction with thanks to my teachers, *Bachmann* and *de la Fuye,* who shall always have my deep respect. My thanks also go to my friends and collaborators in word and deed, especially *Feucht,* for perusal of the first, German-language version. I am grateful to the publishers for the fine layout and publication. And special thanks go to my wife, who not only helped me in my acupuncture studies, but whose constructive criticism has given me much initiative, also in regard to this book.

Chapter I

THE SIMPLEST FORMS OF ACUPUNCTURE AND THE POINTS THEY REQUIRE

The Precepts of Acupuncture

The Precepts of Acupuncture: Right at the beginning of this book, I would like to quote my teacher, *de la Fuye,* who best described the potential and limits of acupuncture: "In acupuncture, gold, silver, or steel needles are inserted into exactly determined points on the skin, which are spontaneously sensitive or sensitive to pressure, in functional, reversible illnesses or disorders for therapeutic and/or diagnostic purposes." When this definition is divided into its individual parts, the result is the step-by-step structure of this book, as well as that of acupuncture itself. Since this therapeutic method is one of the oldest medical methods still used today, we may assume that it originally developed from using pressure or gentle massage on a painful spot to alleviate pain. Every mother still does this to her child today, and one does it oneself – one could say as an instinctive reflex.

Primitive Acupuncture or Locus-Dolendi-Needling

Primitive Acupuncture or Locus-Dolendi-Needling: This procedure is still very widespread throughout Eastern Asia. It is usually done by laymen on the street and does not require a great degree of knowledge. The needle is inserted into the painful locus (usually no deeper than 4-20 mm) and removed again either immediately or after only a few minutes. The alleviative effect is usually immediate, however, not always very long-lasting. Today, we also use this method occasionally, especially for local muscle cramps, such as those quite often afflicting athletes. This type of needling is also often used for the most varying types of pain, however, only to achieve a supplementary action.

The alert human mind soon observed that certain types of pain always corresponded to the same painful areas on the skin. These skin points were recorded, catalogued as to their topography and indication, and soon, an index of these points, which always appeared in certain illnesses, was compiled. Acupuncture having originated in ancient China, the points were given descriptive names, which we no longer need to memorize today.

Master Points

Master Points: The points which proved to be especially effective in the treatment of certain diseases or painful conditions, were called master points. Since the exact differentiation of pathological conditions was still unknown at that time, these master points were given the name of the organ or functional group upon which they had the most influence. Therefore, today we still speak of a master point of the stomach, a master point of the musculature, of the diaphragm, etc. These master points were used in all illnesses in which the corresponding organ or function was disturbed, without the specific pathological process having been taken into consideration. That means, they were, and still are today, acupunctured no matter whether **hypo**secretion of the stomach, for example, or **hyper**secretion is being dealt with. This master point of the stomach lies 2 fingerbreadths lateral to the dorsal midline on both sides of the body (that is, on the left and on the right) between the transverse processes of the 12th thoracic and 1st lumbar vertebrae. In every patient suffering from a stomach ailment, regardless of the specific type, the pain will be transmitted to this area. Normally, the patient is unable to pinpoint the exact locus himself, but, if the area is explored with a bougie or similar instrument, he will very quickly indicate a precise punctiform skin zone measuring up to 5 mm in diameter. This point can now be massaged with the finger or an instrument; a cupping-glass can be applied to it; impletol (a local anesthetic) can be injected, or a needle simply inserted. After a short interval, the patient will always report a change in his condition.

Obviously, cutaneous-visceral reflexes are at work. Eastern literature in particular likes to treat acupuncture as a target cutaneous reflex therapy, which it no doubt is. However, later we will see that there is more to it. Of course, one can also evaluate the diagnostic value only of these points. If, in keeping with the example above, the patient reports spontaneous pain in the region in question, which increases when the actual point is touched, then we know that a stomach disorder is present. But, with our present knowledge, which is limited to the master points, we are unable to give any further details as to the specific type of disorder with which we are dealing.

Symptomatic Points

Symptomatic Points: In the course of time, a large number of points were found which did not have such a general influence on the organs, but produced better results in certain illnesses either by themselves or combined with other points, including the master points. The total number of all points is said to be about 750. Of course, in daily practice one does by no means need all of them. This applies especially to the beginner. For him, only the most important, always applicable points shall be presented here. Every physician is familiar with some of these points anyway, for example, Valleix's points. These have the same diagnostic value in acupuncture, but also serve target therapy at the same time. Here, the difference in the evaluation of sensitive skin points in our medicine and in Chinese medicine is particularly obvious. These points often have only one specific action; sometimes several; their action is rarely wide-range. However, this applies only if they are used alone. Usually, a combination of several points is used to achieve a certain result. This is valid not only for therapy, but for diagnosis as well.

Allow me to give you an example. But first, I must explain that in order to bring clarity into the myriad of points, a special nomenclature is employed. All points lie on paths of conduction, which are called meridians, and which will be discussed in more detail later. Their names will then be given in abbreviated form, and each individual point thereof is given a number. This facilitates orientation. Here, however, I shall still describe the location, as the meridians and the numeration have not yet been discussed.

Let us assume that a patient suffers from headaches and we want to find the cause. We have roughly the following possibilities: We look for a point which lies half a fingerbreadth cranial to the middle of the cheek bone (os zygomaticum). If this point is very sensitive to pressure, we have to consider either a hormonal component (especially in women), sinusitis or vasomotor rhinitis, or vertigo as being the cause. The point has the abbreviated name G 3. Now, if a point on the lower end of the occipital bone on the dorsal midline (PV 16) and a point in the middle of the first sacral foramen (B 31) are also sensitive, we can narrow the cause down to a hormonal component. However, if both these points are insensitive, we must examine a point on the ventral midline, 2 fingerbreadths below the navel. If this point (CV 6) and the point on the temple (G 3) are painful, we must assume that vascular vertigo is the cause of the headaches. However, if these points are not markedly altered, we must test points over the supraorbital foramen (B 2) or on the cranial end of the nasolabial groove (LI 20). If these points are very sensitive, vasomotor rhinitis or sinusitis is the cause of this cephalaea. Other causes can be found in a similar manner. I shall describe these later on.

Now we can treat the patient with acupuncture or any other suitable method. At any rate, we can be quite sure of achieving our therapeutic aim without taking any detours. In addition, these points may be located and examined very rapidly. Of course, we can also use the above-mentioned points therapeutically when indicated by simply inserting a suitable needle. Combinations like these shall be repeatedly mentioned. They are not, however, meant to be used indiscriminately.

The Energetic Pilot Points

The Energetic Pilot Points: First, several concepts must be explained. The concept of energy continuously circulating in the body in set pathways (meridians) is new to us. This concept has been handed down by the ancient Chinese and must be maintained at least in the beginning as a working hypothesis for it has proven to be most effective in practice. In order to explain the following facts, the Chinese used their philosophical concepts, thus transforming the – then still empirical medicine – or acupuncture – into a science. The concept was as follows: Two forces which maintain life are distinguished. These are the so-called YANG and YIN, the philosophical polarities, like light and dark, hot and cold, day and night, man and woman, etc. They act simultaneously in the body and are antagonists at the same time.

Complete balance of these two forces maintains perfect health. Thus, they can be compared to he terms sympathetic and parasympathetic, or better, adrenergic and cholinergic (as these erms also contain an energetic concept). These two factors, YANG and YIN, are components of the so-called life energy, TSRI, which is defined as the sum of and prerequisite for all manifestations of life.

Maintaining this energy and achieving the best possible balance of its two main components, YANG and YIN, is the dominating element of ancient Chinese medicine. In the beginning, we find this concept of an energetic process unusual. However, it leads us directly into the dynamic field of all physiological and pathological processes which are so difficult to comprehend. The fact that energy of this kind exists and is vital does not stand to question, because, after all, we always operate using the terms power of resistance, strong reactions, etc., even though these factors cannot be easily measured, at least not in daily practice. From physics and chemistry we know the different forms energy can take, as well as its potential for transformation, whereby release and deficit of energy in chemical processes are the most common. However, in transferring the concept of energy to the human body, we are forced to think not in terms of small cell groups, but in terms of the whole condition. According to the acknowledged basic laws of chemistry, matter cannot be gained, nor can it be lost, therefore, in a homogenous organism, losses or gains of individual parts must be at the cost or to the benefit of other parts.

This coincides with the ancient Chinese view that there can be no single isolated illness. Therefore, their therapy aims at reinstating the normal (vegetative) equilibrium, which has been disturbed by an illness in one organ followed by the attempt of all systems to achieve physiological regulation. In keeping with the Oriental way of thinking, all perceptions were put into metaphors. Thus, energy is compared with water which flows continuously through certain channels (meridians) and, if necessary, can be directed into other channels or held there by means of sluices (the still to be discussed energetic pilot points). This comparison is very vivid and can be utilized as a working hypothesis, because acupuncture wants nothing more than to correctly distribute the existing energy, if the body is incapable of doing so itself.

At this point, I must interject that we of the "Vienna School of Acupuncture" use the concept of energy mainly as a working hypothesis. We, ourselves, base our work rather on pathophysiology and physiology. In spite of the differing ways of approaching the problem of point selection, both ways lead as a rule to the same point combinations. It can therefore be said that acupuncture performed in adherence to the ancient, traditional rules still works today.

Chapter II

ENERGY AND THE MERIDIANS

I have already briefly mentioned the energy, TSRI, and established that it consists of two components, YANG and YIN. These two concepts shall accompany us throughout the entire discussion of energetic acupuncture, that is, the higher level of this method. We could replace these terms with adrenergic and cholinergic, but it would soon become necessary to continually elaborate on these terms in connection with individual cases, which would only cause confusion. Therefore, it seems imperative to retain these terms, if for no other reason than because they are used in all standard works on acupuncture and in some respects far surpass our more confined synonyms.

Sources of Energy

Sources of Energy: There are various sources of energy. First, there is a general life energy, which is given to each newborn child by its parents. In the Western world, we call this constitution, intelligence, habitus, and hereditary factors. In humans, this is taken for granted; in animal-breeding, great value is placed on these factors. The ancient Chinese as well took this into consideration especially as they could keep several wives and thus pass on a variety of hereditary factors all under the same family name.

Other sources of energy are common to both cultures. These include nutrition, breathing, external influences, etc., however, these factors were evaluated differently by the Chinese, who distinguish, for example, YANG foods and YIN foods, corresponding approximately to our concepts of anabolic and catabolic calories. This also explains the discrepancy between the quantitatively small food consumption and the amount of physical work performed by the average Chinese population in comparison to the ratio in the West.

However, other sources of energy, such as the so-called cosmic energy, are new to us. As realists, we find such expressions suspicious. However, we can easily comprehend them as changes in the electrical fields of force on the earth. I will briefly discuss this later with reference to scientific studies. Here, I would like to add that the Chinese are definitely not a mystical people. On the contrary, they are decided realists. However, they have long understood how to accomplish certain things on earth with the use of higher forces. For example, when a house was constructed, geomancers were called upon to find out whether various spirits would be pleased with the foreseen location of the building. In reality, these people were talented landscape architects and were responsible for the beauty and organic structure of the Chinese scenery and villages, which can still be seen today. Nevertheless, the prospective builders would surely not have taken a "human" suggestion seriously. By the way, in respect to many things in life, we are no different.

Another source of energy is the so-called intersexual energy. This is a certain state of tension when people of opposite sexes meet. I mean the phenomenon which can be seen when several bored men are sitting in a train compartment. The picture changes dramatically when a female enters – she need not be pretty or young. One can actually see the energy flow in these men; their posture changes, etc. This example, which is also valid vice-versa, seems to me to illustrate best the concept of intersexual energy.

No matter from which source the energy is taken, the energy used must be replaced, the sum always remaining constant. A reduction leads to degeneration, and consequently to death. According to the views of the Chinese, the available energy circulates in set, closed pathways.

The Meridians

The Meridians: The name we use for these pathways is a poor translation. The original expression was Kings. There are 12 of these meridians or Kings, and energy circulates therein constantly in a set rhythm, whereby each meridian is in a maximum state for two hours per day. The 12 meridians are arranged in pairs, that means, like mirror images on the left and right side of the body. Each meridian (or King) corresponds with an organ or functional group. These 12 meridians are again divided into 6 YANG meridians and 6 YIN meridians. However, this does not mean that only YANG or YIN energy components flow through them respectively, rather, this designation depends on the functions of the organ to which they correspond. In this way, YANG disorders and YIN disorders are distinguished. One could also say, the disorders result from an excess (YANG) or deficiency (YIN), from hyperfunction (YANG) or hypofunction (YIN). These pathways are the paths of conduction for the circulation of energy, whereby it must be stressed that this is not equivalent to blood circulation, which, by the way, was known to the Chinese long before Harvey.

The Circulation of Energy

The Circulation of Energy: The energy circulates through the body in a sequence like that of the meridians. In the following table, I have taken the fact into consideration that later on, the points lying on the meridians shall be referred to with their abbreviated names. The meridians' names, the abbreviations thereof, and so-called maximum times are as follow.

Meridian	English	German	French	No.	Maximum Time
Heart	H	H	C	I	12:00 noon - 2:00 PM
Small Intestine	SI	Dü(D)	IG	II	2:00 - 4:00 PM
Bladder	B (Bl)	B	V	III	4:00 - 6:00 PM
Kidney	K (Ki)	N	R	IV	6:00 - 8:00 PM
Pericardium (Envelope of the Heart)	P	KS	ECS(MdC)	V	8:00 - 10:00 PM
Triple Heater	3H (TrH) (TrW)	3E	TrR	VI	10:00 PM - 12:00 midnight
Gallbladder	G (GB)	G (B)	Vb	VII	12:00 midnight - 2:00 AM
Liver	Li	Le	F	VIII	2:00 - 4:00 AM
Lung	Lu	Lu	P	IX	4:00 - 6:00 AM
Large Intestine	LI	Di (D)	GI	X	6:00 - 8:00 AM
Stomach	St	M	E	XI	8:00 - 10:00 AM
Spleen-Pancreas	SP	MP	RP	XII	10:00 AM - 12:00 noon
Conception Vessel (Jenn-Mo)	CV	KG (JM)	VC	XIII	————
Pilot Vessel (Tou-Mo)	PV (GV)	LG (GG)	VG	XIV	————

In the table above, the different abbreviations in each language have also been taken into consideration, thus, for example, 3H or TrH(W); or in German, Dü or DüD. The Roman numeration depends on whether we have the circulation begin in the classical manner with the Meridian of the Heart, or with daybreak (dawn) (the Meridian of the Lung). The maximum time corresponds approximately to local time, but can vary slightly. During these hours, the meridians can be maximally influenced. The last two vessels under the triple line of course will surprise you. Up to now, I have only spoken of 12 meridians; now, all of a sudden there are 14 on the list. As you may infer from the description, the last two are not meridians at all, but rather, they are the only two single "extraordinary vessels" which require mention here, as many important points lie thereupon. They shall be dealt with in detail later on.

The First Cycle of Energy

The First Cycle of Energy: We now turn to the topographic course of the meridians. We call a succession of 4 meridians a cycle because that is what they actually form as you will see. The first meridian of the first cycle is the Meridian of the Heart. It begins on the lateral wall of the chest and travels to the fingers (to the fifth or small finger). The Meridian of the Heart is a YIN meridian and as such travels along the inner, or volar, side of the extremity. This rule is also a valuable study aid: All YIN meridians travel along the inner or volar side of the extremities. All YANG meridians travel along the outer or dorsal side. Mnemonically: YANG ... outer, YIN ... inner.

The energy goes from the finger into the next meridian, the Meridian of the Small Intestine (a YANG meridian) along the outer side of the upper extremity to the shoulder. From there, it travels to the head, to the earlobe. From the head, the energy flows into the Meridian of the Bladder (again a YANG meridian), over the back (the course of this meridian is somewhat more complicated, having two neighboring paths), along the dorsolateral side of the leg to the toes (to the fifth or small toe). From there, the energy goes to the Meridian of the Kidney (a YIN meridian) over the inner, or volar, side of the lower extremity and the torso back to the wall of the chest. (Here, the meridian ends somewhat atypically on the sternoclavicular joint). Therewith, the first cycle is closed.

The order YIN-YANG-YANG-YIN is interesting. After each two meridians in the table, a line has been drawn. This means that these two meridians have a special relationship (to be discussed later). We call them partner meridians or partner organs. When a specific point is acupunctured, they can exchange energy internally. However, this exchange can only take place when the energy content in the partner meridians is quantitatively and qualitatively different.

On account of the different courses on the outer or inner side of the extremities, the beginning and end points of the meridians are more or less remote. This makes continuity in the flow of energy seem impossible. In such cases, the connection is maintained by so-called secondary vessels. You will find these secondary vessels again in the discussion of the reunion points. In keeping with our figurative comparison with water, these may be seen as rivulets, like local diversion canals in dams.

The Second Cycle of Energy

The Second Cycle of Energy: This cycle also has the same basic sequence: lateral wall of the chest – finger, finger – head, head – toes, toes – lateral wall of the chest. It starts with the Pericardium Meridian, or Envelope of the Heart. It is a YIN meridian and thus travels from the lateral wall of the chest along the inner side of the upper extremity (radial to the Meridian of the Heart), this time to the middle, or 3rd, finger. It serves two different, and yet similar, functions. From the fingers (here from the ring, or 4th, finger), the energy travels dorsally as a YANG meridian over the hand and arm to the shoulder and on to the tragus of the ear. This meridian is called the Triple Heater (or Triple Warmer). Its name sounds foreign and unscientific to us, but it is easy to remember and describes its function well. This is a purely functional meridian, not directly corresponding to an organ of its own. It reflects the functions of the respiratory, digestive, and urogenital tracts and has a favorable influence both on the individual functions as well as on their interaction. Furthermore, the action on individual organs and their functions may be intensified via this meridian. For example, if we are confronted with a disorder in the respiratory tract, we can treat it directly via the Meridian of the Lung, or we can approach this disorder with the Triple Heater Meridian at the same time. The same also applies to the other corresponding functional groups, the action thereby being intensified. Again, these two organs are partners, just as the Heart and Small Intestine, and the Bladder and Kidney are.

The meridian that now follows, that of the Gallbladder (a YANG meridian), begins again on the head (lateral to the orbit of the eye) and travels, roughly-drawn, laterally along the anterior side of the torso, and then strictly laterally over the lower extremity to the dorsal side of the foot, ending on the 4th toe. From there, the energy flows into the Meridian of the Liver (beginning on the big toe), a YIN meridian, over the inner side of the lower extremity and ventrally along the torso and back again to the lateral wall of the chest. Now the second cycle is closed. Again we see a very similar course: again, the sequence YIN-YANG-YANG-YIN; again, two partner organs. The maximum times, which may be confirmed especially regarding the Meridian of the Gallbladder (12:00 midnight to 2:00 AM), are of interest.

The Third Cycle of Energy

The Third Cycle of Energy: We find the same pattern here. The Meridian of the Lung (a YIN meridian) begins on the lateral wall of the chest, travels from there along the inner side of the upper extremity, however, this time, absolutely radially, downwards, and ends on the thumb. Because its maximum time is from 4:00 to 6:00 AM, that is, coincides with dawn, some authors start the meridians' sequence with the Meridian of the Lung. It is followed by the Meridian of the Large Intestine, which begins on the second, or index, finger, travels dorsally over the back of the hand and arm, and ends on the head (on the upper end of the nasolabial groove). It is a YANG meridian, and is therefore followed by another YANG meridian, the Meridian of the Stomach. This meridian begins laterally on the head, travels approximately along the mamillary line over the torso, and mediolaterally down the leg, ending on the second toe. From there, the energy finally returns via the Meridian of the Spleen-Pancreas (noteworthy is the fact that the Chinese classified these two organs, which are supplied by the same artery, as belonging together already at that time). The Meridian of the Spleen-Pancreas is a YIN meridian. It begins on the big toe and travels along the inner side of the lower extremity and the abdomen back to the lateral wall of the chest, where it end on the 6th intercostal space. From here the energy again passes into the Meridian of the Heart and the circulation with its three respective cycles begins anew. Thus, the circulation of energy appears to be closed, at least in regard to its theoretical structure.

Studies on the Meridians

Studies on the Meridians: At this point, several questions arise. First: Can the meridians, with their sometimes bizarre courses, as seen on charts, be scientifically verified? On the basis of the data available to date, the question must be answered in the negative. A histological substratum of the meridians (contrary to the points) has not yet been demonstrated. On the other hand, the meridians demonstrate distinctly reduced electrical skin resistance, even if to a lesser extent than the points do. Some meridians (for example, the Meridian of the Heart) correspond entirely to typical courses of pain radiation (angina pectoris); others correspond partially (such as sciatic pain on a portion of the Bladder Meridian and sometimes of the Gallbladder Meridian as well). This leads us to studies by *Lang* and *Quaglia-Senta*, who regard the meridians as a chain of receptors and compare them with other systems. In my opinion, the meridians may consist of boundary surfaces of embryonic segments. However, no exact studies thereupon have yet been done. *Mann* was the only one to study the Meridian of the Gallbladder in particular and to suggest a connection with the lateral line organ in fish.

However, at times, the meridians are clearly revealed. As a beginner, I had just such an experience. This was very important for me since I had just become familiar with the meridians and was sceptical as to their existence and courses, and only acknowledged the points. At that time, there was absolutely no scientific foundation for acupuncture, and, as a surgeon, it was hard for me to trust such a method. The following happened: I had known an elderly lady of over 60 for more than 30 years. She had always been completely deaf and was unable to perceive sound even with a hearing aid. Therefore, she had always had to read lips. Even as a boy I was fascinated with this woman's special sensitivity even though I could not explain it. Just after I had started studying acupuncture, I visited her, as she had moved out of the city in the meantime. During a long conversation, she complained of various maladies, as is usual in the company of a physician. Her main complaint was pain in the lower extremities. Let me add that the main point for all pain, particularly in the lower extremities, is the point Bladder Meridian 60 (B 60). It lies on the upper edge of the calcaneum halfway between the external malleolus and the Achilles tendon. I must also add that the Meridian of the Bladder has a seemingly odd bend at the calf. I already carried needles with me at that time, which was certainly premature for a beginner, and briefly told her about my new studies, as acupuncture was still completely unknown in Austria at that time. I then inserted a needle in the above-mentioned point on this woman upon which she said that she felt "something," which travelled through her body in a most unique way. Upon my request to show me where she felt this sensation, she drew the exact course of the Bladder Meridian – it is the longest meridian and has branches – on her own body. I was most impressed and then tried out all the other meridians on this ideal test subject by inserting a needle in the appropriate point of every respective meridian. This woman drew the exact course of each meridian on her body every single time.

The only explanation for this phenomenon is that persons who have been denied one of their senses for a longer period of time are able to employ other, probably more primitive, receptors. Of course, this depends on the person's sensitivity in general, just as observed in particular sensitivity on acupuncture points. *Helen Keller* is an example. She was deaf and blind, but with the exceptionally sensitive palms of her hands into which all words were spelled, she was able to earn two doctorates. *Szillard* once presented color photographs in which he was able to capture partial and, less frequently, total meridian courses in the form of pronounced dermography after acupuncture of individual points on his Hungarian patients. However, the majority of patients do not perceive these meridian courses, but they do feel the individual points.

Hence, we have established that there is electrophysical and functional evidence of the existence of the meridians. However, they have not yet been verified histologically.

The Function of the Meridians

The Function of the Meridians: Aside from the transport of energy which has been thoroughly discussed, all important acupuncture points lie on the meridians. Because of the fact that these points are often used not for regulation, but rather, according to the symptoms to which they correspond, they must also be able to be comprehended accordingly in relation to the meridians. Contrarily, the meridians must also have criteria which relate them to the points lying thereupon. Therefore, when speaking of a meridian, we must not think solely of the organ after which it is named, but rather, also of the points lying thereon and used according to symptomatology. Therefore, we distinguish according to the main action:

1. Meridian of the Heart	distinct influence on the psyche
2. Meridian of the Small Intestine	acts spasmolytically and on the mucous membrane
3. Meridian of the Bladder	the meridian of elimination
4. Meridian of the Kidney	the meridian of dissimilation; also influences the circulation via the adrenal gland
5. Pericardium Meridian (Envelope of the Heart)	for circulatory and sexual symptoms
6. Meridian of the Triple Heater	supports the respiratory, digestive, and urogenital functions
7. Meridian of the Gallbladder	psychological and spasmolytic influence
8. Meridian of the Liver	the meridian of assimilation
9. Meridian of the Lung	respiratory tract; effective for all types of congestion
10. Meridian of the Large Intestine	acts on the mucous membrane; meridian of elimination
11. Meridian of the Stomach	psychologically stabilizing as well as effective for digestion and circulation
12. Meridian of the Spleen-Pancreas	main meridian of connective tissue

In addition, we have the two vessels mentioned above which are not meridians and are not included in the regular circulation of energy, but on which many important points are located.

13. Conception Vessel or JENN-MO. Its course is that of the ventral midline. Its action is somatic in general on regional functions, that is, in the abdominal area, on urogenital and digestive activity, and influences the lungs and heart in the thoracic region.
14. Pilot or Governor Vessel or TOU-MO. Its course is that of the dorsal midline. Its lower portions act somatically, especially on the urogenital tract, its upper portions rather influencing the psyche.

These latter two vessels are of course not partners.

Another question that arises regarding the meridians is, "How can the supply of energy in the individual meridians be determined, and how and when can or must it be regulated?" This shall be dealt with later on.

Chapter III

THE DIFFERENT TYPES OF POINTS

Main and Special Points: The points that we will discuss now are used to properly distribute energy or balance energetic discrepancies. One could also say that we use them to combat the above-mentioned YANG and YIN disorders. In each meridian, we distinguish 2 main points and 4 special points, these having different functions. Let's begin with the main points.

Main and Special Points

The Tonification Point: This point always lies on the meridian to which it belongs. If there is an energy deficiency in its meridian (and thus in its corresponding organ or function), it sends energy to it. We call this conveyance of energy tonification. In general, a tonification point is acupunctured with a gold needle because the Chinese attribute tonifying qualities to gold and all other "yellow" metals. The tonification point can also be used purely symptomatically. In acupuncture, an either-or situation is very rare. Rather, one must regard it as a manifold phenomenon. Hence, it is perfectly feasible that a tonification point be used only as a locus dolendi point one time; another time, solely on the basis of symptoms, and finally, in advanced acupuncture, as a tonification point for regulation of the flow of energy.

The Tonification Point

The Sedation Point: This point as well always lies on the meridian to which it belongs. If there is an excess of energy in its meridian, it directs energy away from it. We call this removal of energy sedation. In general, a sedation point is acupunctured with a silver needle as the Chinese attribute sedation qualities to silver and all other "white" metals. The comments stated above regarding the varying usage of the tonification point apply here as well. It must also be stressed that a sedation point's list of symptoms mainly contains conditions which require sedation. The opposite is true of tonification points.

The Sedation Point

Let us now turn to the so-called special points.

The Source Point: This point is an adjuvant to the respective main point. That means, its manner of action depends on which main point is administered at the same time and (according to the Chinese) on the metal of the needles inserted into these two combined points.

The Source Point

In practice, this means that, for example, in the case of a greater energy deficiency, the tonification point alone is inadequate or is unable to counteract the meridian's energetic deficit fast enough. The source point is then used simultaneously and enhances and expediates the tonification point's action. The same of course also applies to the opposite indication, an overabundance of energy. Here, the sedation point of the appropriate meridian and its source point are acupunctured simultaneously. For sedation, both points are acupunctured with silver needles; for tonification, both with gold needles.

Thus, the source point is basically ambivalent and the direction of its action depends only on the simultaneously administered main point and the metal of the needles used.

The Passage or Lo Point: This point's manner of action is somewhat more difficult to explain. Although this point always lies on the meridian to which it belongs, its action also extends to another meridian, which we call its partner meridian. I refer you to the previous discussion of the meridians in regard to the circulation of energy and to the line after each pair of meridians in the table. Here, we always find one YANG and one YIN meridian as partners. They follow each other in the circulation of energy, however not in the sequence 1 and 2, 2 and 3, 3 and 4, etc., but rather in the sequence 1 and 2, 3 and 4, 5 and 6 etc. In other words, there is no consecutive connection between the meridians, but rather, the connection is that of pairs. These individual pairs have particular qualities and special relationships, which shall be dealt with again later.

The Passage or Lo Point

An internal energy exchange so to speak can take place via the passage or Lo point of one or the other of the partner meridians. The passage point is used when one meridian has an abundance of energy, but its partner has an energy deficiency. In general, the diversion takes place from the meridian rich in energy to the meridian lacking energy, however there are also opposing views on this. We adhere to the following: If partner meridians have different energy conditions, we "save" needles via the passage point. Otherwise, we would have to acupuncture the sedation point in the strong meridian and perhaps also the source point, and in the weak meridian, the tonification point and perhaps also the source point. We can achieve the same results with one needle in the passage point of one – as already said, usually stronger – meridian.

The Alarm or Herald Point

The Alarm or Herald Point: This is another special point. It can, but does not necessarily, lie on the meridian to which it belongs. Some meridians have more than one alarm or herald point. It is usually spontaneously sensitive, often actually painful, not only in acute disorders, as its name implies, but even more so, in chronic disorders of a meridian or organ to which the meridian particularly corresponds. Whenever it is spontaneously sensitive, it should be included in the treatment, and it also has significant diagnostic value for those who intend to utilize acupuncture's concepts solely for diagnosis.

The Associated or Concurring ("Assentiment"*) Point

The Associated or Concurring ("Assentiment"*) Point: No matter to which meridian or corresponding organ it may be ascribed, this point always lies on the Meridian of the Bladder, that is, on its first course along the spine, approximately 2 fingerbreadths lateral to the dorsal midline and between the two transverse processes of neighboring vertebrae. These points most closely approach our segmental way of thinking. They are of great value both diagnostically and therapeutically, for acute as well as chronic illnesses in particular, and as a supplement to the sedation points. They shall be discussed in more detail later.

Now that we have discussed the main and special points, let us turn to other extraordinary points.

The Reunion Point

The Reunion Point: Via cross-connections, these points have the capacity to connect several meridians (and therewith, several functions) and achieve a mutual action. With these points, a significantly more extensive action on disturbed functions and functional complexes may be achieved. Just as with the passage point, one is able to keep the number of simultaneously used needles down to a minimum, thus making the treatment more agreeable for the patient. They are somewhat more difficult to use for differential diagnosis, especially for the beginner. It is considered practically a technical error if they are not included in the treatment when found to be spontaneously sensitive.

Here, I would like to use two reunion points as an example. We find the most important point for the treatment of cervical syndrome and cervical migraine on the dorsal midline on the tip of the spinal process of the 7th cervical vertebra. This is the point PV 13. The point CV 15, the point for treatment of Roemheld's syndrome, lies on the ventral midline just distal to the tip of the xiphoid.

The point PV 13 is also called the "spider". Cross-connections, the so-called secondary vessels, proceed from this point to a series of points. Drawn on a diagram of the neck, the result looks like a spider sitting in the middle of its web.

The points which are directly connected with PV 13 are: PV 16, B 10, G 20, 3H 15, LI 15, SI 9, B 39.

Therefore, instead of acupuncturing each of these points individually, we can replace them all with PV 13.

---

*)borrowed from the French

However, if stress is to be laid on a certain influential factor or indication of one of the respective connected points, we can by all means include that point. For example: cervical migraine with strong susceptibility to weather influences, radiating to the frontal region of the head: Combination: PV 13, 3H 15, 3H 22, 3H 17, B 2, PdM, G 14.

The Cardinal Point

The Cardinal Point: Again, a small introduction is necessary. These points are connection points of the so-called "extraordinary vessels or MOs." In keeping with the previously used comparison of energy with a regulated flow of water, these represent reservoirs so to speak, with which energy can be quickly redistributed in extreme cases of poor energy regulation. The cardinal points represent the connecting mechanisms of this advanced form of acupuncture. Because of the fact that even in the above example, spontaneous, rapid, energetic changes may be expected, the beginner is warned against ever acupuncturing a cardinal point first or last in a point combination. Because, if there is no emergency, and one does not possess great practical experience, but still sets abrupt and vehement energetic processes like these into motion, acupuncture, which is otherwise completely harmless, can sometimes call forth a blockage, and in any case, jeopardize the success of the treatment. However, one can of course include these points symptomatically in an acupuncture point combination without running the risk of causing injurious side-effects.

Points Outside of the Meridians and Personal Points

Points Outside of the Meridians and Personal Points: There are also several points which do not lie on the paths of conduction, or meridians. They shall be dealt with according to their significance in the discussion of the most important points. These points are ever-present, but have nothing directly to do with the regulation of energy. According to the information available at present, especially from *Petricek* and *Zeitler,* they are considered as satellite points. The nomenclature developed by the above authors seems logical as well as practical. If a point with the same or similar indications lies on the same meridian near a known point (for example, St 36), it is called 36-1 or 2, 3, 4, etc. depending on its proximity to the meridian point. If the satellite point lies outside the meridian (medial or lateral to it), but corresponds either partially or entirely to it, its name is also dependent on its proximity to the meridian point, i.e. St 36-01, 02, 03, 04, etc. With this terminology (which is most closely related to subsequent computer compilation) the reader is spared the separate study of the so-called "new points, points outside the meridians, extra points, 'points curieux', etc."

Personal points are a different matter. They only appear on certain individuals and then, only temporarily. When revealed, they should always be included in the treatment. If they disappear after the treatment, prognostically favorable conclusions can be made.

Thus, we have again come full circle, starting with the most primitive form of acupuncture, inserting a needle into a painful point, to the symptomatic use of selected points, to the regulation of energy via the main and special points; from the complex method of treatment with the reunion points, and the emergency regulation of energy by means of the cardinal points, back to the primitive personal points.

Before I present evidence and research results regarding the above, I would like to stress again that the best proof of any method is reliable efficiency in practice. And because this book is meant for practical application, only the most important aspects of the various studies shall be mentioned.

Research on Various Acupunctural Phenomena

Research on Various Acupunctural Phenomena: Ever since acupuncture became known in the West there have been attempts either to confirm or reject it. The acupuncture point was always the center of attention. How does it differ from its surroundings? It differs in various ways. First of all, everybody with some degree of sensitivity has a "different" feeling when certain, relatively small, point-formed spots on the skin are touched in comparison to the sensation when neighboring areas are stimulated. Hence, the same pressure applied with a suitably small instrument is perceived differently on neighboring point-formed areas. The diameter of a point is relatively small, about 3-5 mm, so that palpation with the fingertip can only lead a skilled physician to the point. These points of the skin, whose sensitivity differs from other skin points, were quickly verified as identical to the acupuncture points.

Electrical Measurement of Resistance on Skin Points

Electrical Measurement of Resistance on Skin Points: Because a connection between the skin points and regulation of energy was well known from the classical concepts handed down to us, energy was mainly thought of in terms of electrical energy and attempts were made to examine levels thereof on the points. Indeed, the electrical behavior of these points was different from that of the immediate surrounding skin areas of the same structure. They were shown to be zones of reduced electrical skin resistance and soon, based thereupon, commercial firms constructed measuring devices to locate the points. There are many such instruments, such as those constructed by *de la Fuye, Kindling, Niboyet,* and *Voll,* just to name a few. The latter far surpasses point detection and location in its use, the so-called electro-acupuncture according to *Voll* being based thereupon. This method also uses the concepts and points of classical acupuncture, however, needles are usually not inserted, but rather, the attempt is made to achieve energetic balance on the points by means of an electrical charge or discharge. A more detailed discussion of this method would go beyond our present frame of reference, especially as other persons are much more qualified to speak on this subject than I.

In measuring these points, a dot electrode is applied to the skin portion in question by the examiner, while the patient holds a second electrode in his hand. Systematically, the point electrode is repeatedly applied to the skin so that one measurement area after the other is established. When the point has been exactly located, the indicator drops in some instruments; other devices have a magic eye or give a signal. These devices are suited for the beginner as they free him from the fear of not finding the point he is looking for and help him to learn the points' positions. Furthermore, they act as a control for those doing research. For example, the points used in the studies by the Viennese histologist, *Kellner,* which I shall describe later, were established in advance with devices of this type designed by *Feucht.*

The difficulties inherent in measurements such as these should not go unmentioned. In particular, the varying dampness on different parts of the skin, which is also the result of a longer examination period, can cause variations or changes. Secondly, we have the varying application pressure of the electrodes used by the examiner. Attempts were made to eliminate both factors by drying or even moistening the area to be examined and constructing detection electrodes with pressure constants. Measuring electrical skin resistance is difficult, but in practice, acquisition of exact values is much less important because the reduction on the acupuncture point is so marked that it is revealed in any case.

We may summarize by saying that acupuncture points can be located with measuring devices. They are approached as small areas of reduced electrical skin resistance. Accordingly, they differ distinctly from the areas surrounding them.

Electrically Superior Points of the Skin

Electrically Superior Points of the Skin: This term was coined by the Viennese physicist, *Maresch,* who also established specific electrical behavior on single, tiny skin areas in studies on the susceptibility of humans to weather conditions and changes. He measured atmospheric electricity potentials with the Benndorf electrometer. In undetermined weather conditons, he found considerable electrical unrest in the atmospheric electrical field – in which, of course, the human moves about, and in which an adult of normal height is exposed to a tension of about 200 Volts. This was recognized as a result of changes in humidity (irregular changes in the humidity content of the various atmospheric layers) and an inversion (i.e. a change in the common phenomenon of temperature dropping with increasing height. In the case of inversion, this can be reduced or even reversed). The entire field of atmospheric electricity is altered by these two factors. Therefore, they can also be regarded physically as electric generators. If an individual is susceptible to weather conditions or changes, receptors must exist which respond to the changed electrical conditions. These are located in particular in the skin. The study of the skin was carried out with an oscillograph, a square wave voltage generator and two body electrodes, so that two current curves were presented in constant units of time. The first curve had the values 25 kiloohms and 0.1 microfarads; the second, 50 kiloohms and 0.5 microfarads. These values were also compared to a phantom having ohmic resistance connected to a condensor in series (that is, the basic diagram of connections of the skin). Alterations in both these standard curves were seen on the skin, whereby areas could be established which showed a different electrical behavior than other neighboring, also tiny, areas. These altered curves allow the conclusion that on the loci on the body found by *Maresch*, which were considered electrically superior points of the skin, a substratum must exist which can be regarded as decisive or responsible for these changes. There seems to be a stimulus blockage, this being of great significance for the explanation of weather susceptibility and interesting in its similarity to the behavior of surface-active substances under similar conditions of electrical measurement. Especially important is the fact that the electrical quantities used as well as those measured were congruous with biological quantities.

Summary: Disturbances in the field of atmospheric electricity on certain small areas of the skin can cause measurable and demonstrable changes in electrical values. These points are called electrically superior points of the skin and are congruous with acupuncture points. As these points must be considered receptors, they must possess an according substratum, the structure of which would explain this phenomenon. This leads us to the histology of the acupuncture point. But first, we must become more familiar with the skin as bearer of these points.

The Structure and Function of the Skin

The Structure and Function of the Skin: This is also the title of a fundamental study carried out by the Viennese histologist, *Kellner,* whom I have already quoted ("Bau und Funktion der Haut," Deutsche Zeitschrift für Akupunktur 1, 1966, Karl F. Haug, Heidelberg). I heartily recommend it to anyone interested in the various methods of skin stimulation. Here, I shall only present the most important excerpts. The skin not only has a protective function in the mechanical sense, but is also a means of communication with the environment and a manifold sensory organ. In addition, it participates decisively in the regulation of the entire body. It is equipped for all these tasks with the blood and lymph vessels, as well as the nerves, the *Meissner* corpuscles and end-bulbs of *Krause, Ruffini's* nerve endings, as well as free nerve endings. The basic functions of the skin are performed by its cells whereby their performance again depends on the milieu surrounding them. Furthermore, *Kellner* shows various forms of vascular short circuits, such as the simple arteriovenous anastomoses in their various phases, as well as the *Hoyer-Grosser* or glomus organs, and explains the influence of this regulation of blood flow as an effector action to fill the interstice. Cutaneous fissures which are connected to vessels and smooth muscles, seem to play a decisive role in the swelling process of the papillary body. The types of nerves which supply these muscles are noteworthy. They are adrenergic, myeline, and nonmyelinated nerves having varying courses and end formations. Therefore, they must also be dependent on the surrounding environment. These environment and changes therein will be of great interest again later in the discussion of regulation.

The Histology of the Acupuncture Point

The Histology of the Acupuncture Point: Quite some time ago attempts were already made to differentiate the acupuncture point histologically from the tissue surrounding it using slides on which normal tissue containing a point was mounted. However, no one was ever able to demonstrate a typical substratum and therefore, the dominating opinion was that the acupuncture point had none and that it was at the most a cutaneous projection, or simply did not exist at all. Already at the beginning of my collaboration with *Kellner,* it became obvious that we could not study the acupuncture points in the usual histological manner. Therefore, the extraction of skin matrix on the points, and also on the meridians, and neutral (in regard to acupuncture) skin areas was undertaken for comparison and dissected into 250 to over 300 serial slides. Then, skin matrix with a diameter of 5 to 7 mm was extracted from 24 acupuncture points (and other skin areas) no later than two hours post mortem, prepared and catalogued as mentioned above. The results of these studies were acquired from material consisting of 11, 137 histological slides. Therefore, the danger of error due to insufficient numbers or coincidence was excluded. It was shown that on the acupuncture points – contrary to the meridians and "neutral" skin loci – the number of various nerve endings is significantly increased – also in regard to the composition of different acupuncture points. *Meissner* corpuscles, endbulbs of *Krause,* glomus organs (also called *Hoyer-Grosser* organs), as well as smooth muscle cells were differentiated. These results clearly showed that the acupuncture points are based on a histological substratum, which is capable of the electrophysical activity postulated by *Maresch.*

While these studies were in their initial phase, a book by the North Korean, *Kim Bong Han* appeared on the so-called Kyungrak, or fourth, system. This book contained pictures of unique bodies and pathways which the author interpreted as the substratum of acupuncture points and meridians, although the explanations to the pictures did not always include the customary histological details. *Kellner* had already repeatedly noticed structures of this type in the slides he already had at hand, and this data seemed to make the entire study unnecessary. However, during the examination of the slides under a polarizing microscope – whereby only those slides were selected which were congruous with those published by *Bong Han* – these structures soon proved to be foreign body gigantocytes of talc crystals. Therefore, today we can reject the Kyungrak system as scientifically unfounded. This is also justified for another reason: If all points, and the meridians as well, were based on one and the same substrate, then the various points would not be capable of performing specific actions, or at best, they would be very limited. However, we maintained that there are specific actions, this having been confirmed in daily practice.

Again, we adhere to the following: In specially performed histological examinations, the acupuncture points were shown to be accumulations of end structures with receptor and effector qualities. They differ in type and number in the individual points and therefore allow the assumption that there are different, specific actions with which we are familiar through practical experience. The immediate surrounding area of the otherwise congruous skin zone does not show these accumulations. Therefore, a distinct difference between the point and its surroundings exists. This can be seen particularly in a series of sections which were not absolutely perfect. Here, both parts are seen next to each other on the same slide, however, their respective structures are distinctly different. The so-called Kyungrak system is not a suitable scientific explanation of the acupuncture points.

On the Function of the Skin

On the Function of the Skin: Of course, this is not the place to describe all the skin's functions; only a few characteristics which are associated with acupuncture shall be mentioned here. As already said, only a few punctiform areas of the skin which can be established by sensory means, are inherent in our medicine's methods of examination. These are *Valleix's* points and *Boas'* pressure test points. In my opinion, *McBurney's* point should be included, as well as *Virchow's* node, which is indeed not a point, but can be considered as a test region in cases of cancer of the stomach.

It was rather the reflex zones which have been acknowledged. The hyperalgetic *(Head's)* zones are well known. Although he took *Kellner's* studies into consideration, *Bergsmann* listed other criteria of these zones in his investigations of the skin. Aside from exact inspection, he takes palpation of individual skin parts into particular consideration: Keeping the varying degree of papillary body swelling in mind, this method seems completely logical. Indeed, the skilled acupuncturist is able to verify a point as being a locus in an altered state of swelling through palpation. After successful therapy, the swelling subsides, and the area is once again the same as the surrounding skin in this aspect.

Aside from the changes in the electrical measurement values discussed above, infrared radiation measurement on points and small zones also shows changed values. Likewise, we find changes in type and intensity of the dermography, of artificially produced erythemas, in capillaroscopy of the terminal capillaries, and finally, in the comparison of the number of leukocytes in various sections of the body as well. The latter changes would have to be particularly great in unilateral processes. Phthisiologist *Bergsmann* undertook studies on unilateral pulmonary processes on a series of cases. He discovered distinct differences in the capillary blood of both shoulders in cases of unilateral, specific, and non-specific inflammations of the lungs as well as carcinomas. Under certain circumstances, he also found them analogous, even if in a somewhat weaker form, in blood taken from the fingertip. There were not only quantitative, but also qualitative differences in the white blood count, these providing information on unilateral changes, changes in the flow velocity in the terminal capillaries, and in the capacity of the soft connective tissue, which is so important for regulation. This approaches the laws of acupuncture which recommend that needling be performed on the "healthy" side first in unilateral disorders. These laws seldom allow strictly unilateral treatment (except in cases of unilateral local spasm, etc.) and, as we shall see later on, point out possible transference between meridians of the same name or of energetic components thereof from one side to the other.

Again, we summarize that point-formed, as well as larger, areas exist on the skin which are, or better, become perceptible in different ways when a disturbance of often remote and especially, deeper-lying organs or functions is present. Our medicine makes use thereof for diagnostic purposes only, a one-way street so to speak, while Chinese medicine, especially acupuncture, presupposes and uses the effect on the organ thereby revealing itself via the irritated skin zones as a tool. An experiment done by *Puder* showed that this is both correct and plausible. He did the following experiment on the lungs (pulmonary changes being relatively easy to determine): In animal experiments, strongly irritating substances were repeatedly rubbed into the skin of the thorax producing pneumonic atelecstatic changes in the homolateral lung. At first, one tends to regard embrocation effects of this type as "propagation per continuitatem." However, when the continuity in these experiments was interrupted by producing a pneumothorax, the same changes were seen. The negative effect of other factors which irritate the skin, such as strong insolation, may also correspond.

We have established that proof of the action of skin irritants on deeper-lying organs exists, whereby there was a relative proximity in the case described, making it therefore easier to comprehend.

In the discussion of the various points, we postulated specific, albeit sometimes multiple, actions. The histology of the acupuncture point has revealed its specific structure, which seems to strongly support this postulation. However, we still do not have proof of the specificity of individual points.

Evidence of the Specific Actions of the Individual Points

Evidence of the Specific Actions of the Individual Points: *Bergsmann* again chose the lungs for a very decisive experiment. As we have already seen, the lung is very suitable because of the ease and reliability with which changes therein can be determined. I would like to point out that in tubercular affections of longer standing, particularly caverns, there is a pronounced rigidity of the diaphragm resulting in a reduction of breath volume. Via the point B 17 (2 fingerbreadths paravertebral to the dorsal midline and on both sides between the transverse processes of the 7th and 8th thoracic vertebrae) we have acupuncture's strongest action on the diaphragm at our disposal. In the experiment above, patients were acupunctured on various points, including points of the same segment or region, while under the fluoroscope. No change in the action of the diaphragm took place. But when the point B 17 was acupunctured, distinct excursions were observed which lasted several hours and led to a spirometrically measurable increase of up to 700 cubic centimeters in breathing capacity. These changes were also demonstrable in all cases and could be reproduced again and again.

Now, one could classify this phenomenon as a target cutaneous reflex therapy and therewith reject the regulation we postulated. Thus, this experiment would correspond with that sphere of acupuncture which uses points on the basis of their symptoms and does not delve into the energetic connections which play an integral role in regulation. However, regulative processes must participate here as well, as otherwise there is no explanation for the relatively long-lasting effect and the general and specific improvements observed after repeated needling.

General Comments on Regulation

General Comments on Regulation: First, the concept of regulation needs to be explained. According to *Pischinger's* environmental theory, the primitive vegetative forms of regulation are controlled by a "non-specific basic system," that is, the soft connective tissue and its milieu (which includes the intercellular substance and fluid). Any action on a cell of an organ, be it humoral, hormonal, or neural, must travel through this system. Each organ has its own environment according to its varying specific tasks. A change in the organ can influence the entire environment of the body, as well as that of other organs. Contrarily, it can also be influenced by them.

Therefore, 3 components are distinguished in the vegetative system.

1. a neural component which includes the vegetative-nervous terminal structure,
2. a humoral component which comprises the capillary terminal network, and
3. a component in-between which we call cellular. This includes the reticular stem cells of the soft connective tissue, as well as of the reticulo-endothelial system (R.E.S.); likewise, the intercalary cells according to *Feyrter.*

These three components are very closely related morphologically. They are regulated from three poles, that is, a neural, a humoral, and a neurohormonal. We must consider the nervous terminal structure, the hypophysis and adrenal cortex, the blood, R.E.S., and lymphoid tissue as the means with which this regulation is achieved.

The ability of the entire body to adjust to various interventions can be determined by analysis of the blood picture, iodine consumption tests, sodium and potassium analyses, and also electrical tests. All these tests provide comparable response curves. The acquired curves can be roughly divided into four groups.

1. The so-called normal curve or norm reaction. Here, we see an initial drop in the measured values followed by an increase expressing the onset of counter-regulation.
2. Persistence in the (negative) shock phase.
3. Very rapid onset of counter-reaction. Not only do the values reached remain constant even after a period of hours, but they increase even further, albeit to a lesser extent.
4. The so-called regulative unresponsiveness; that means, the expression of the body's inability to respond to an applied stimulus.

In the discussion of the body's reactions to the needle stimulus, we will again find these four curves. They were already known to the Chinese who considered them the expression of adjustment to a stimulus.

We may summarize by saying that via the milieu, overall regulation, in dependence on three poles of regulation, affects all three constituents of the vegetative system. Four typical forms of regulative response can be determined by a variety of methods, depicted as curves, and observed in clinical practice.

All of the above refers to the general regulation which has become a common term in modern medicine, especially through works by *F. Hoff* and *Selye.* In acupuncture however, we find very specific reactions as well as these general reactions. This means we can bring about exactly determined changes either in the entire body, or in individual parts thereof by needling a precisely determined area of the skin. This goes far beyond reflex therapy. The needle itself reaches the subcutis, this being the intermediate layer between the skin (which we can regard as a boundary surface) and the entire body. Any therapy which is initiated there must necessarily influence this intermediate layer, and therewith convey the stimulus.

Specific Regulation: Studies on the specific regulation were carried out by *Bischko* and *Stacher*. In this experiment, we first tried to determine all disturbing elements. Thus, for example, during a lengthy experiment, we saw that exposure to sunrays could completely alter the measurement values. Comparison with the experimental methods used in the study of general regulation were made. Because blood samples had to be taken from both sides of the body, we were faced with a problem regarding patients with unilateral disorders. Therefore, we soon reverted to measuring skin resistance. Here it was shown that in normal as well as in pathological cases, changes are produced in the skin resistance upon strain, depending on exogenous and endogenous alterations, as well as on the prevailing weather conditions. Here, too, reaction curves were observed which were similar to those common in general regulation. Specific Regulation

In the study, a device for measuring resistance, which was able to derive and register values from six locations was used. All meridians were short-circuited by means of ring electrodes on the wrists and ankles in order to exclude sources of error from the acupuncture points' reduced resistance values. Again, four different measurement curves were observed showing typical reactions, whereby the curve obtained in cases with chronic systematic illnesses was very different to that of healthy subjects. Following an interval, 20 minutes on the average, the resistance in all subjects adjusted to a certain level, and did not change significantly even when the measurements were continued for one hour or more.

When an acupuncture point was needled and the inserted needle connected to the registration and measuring device by means of a clamp during the stabilization phase of the resistance measurement, one of two typical reactions was observed after an initial brief period of unrest:

1. If a point was needled which did not correlate to the subject's disorder or illness in accordance with the laws of acupuncture, then the measurement values did not change; in other words, the curve remained stable.
2. However, if a point significantly corresponding to the existing illness was needled, a very distinct and rapid change in the measurement value took place, and even after a longer period of measurement, the registered values did not return to the levels observed for that particular point prior to insertion of the needle.

We can summarize by saying that it has been proven that a specific change in regulation is produced via the acupuncture points. By means of suitable equipment it was shown that the body can be distinctly influenced in its regulation activities via an indicated point.

Thus, we can consider regulation as a stimulus-dependent process. Therefore, the form regulation takes will depend on the type and intensity of the stimulus. The smallest stimuli are dealt with locally, that is, without the assistance of more complex mechanisms. Stronger stimuli can still be compensated in the periphery by means of reaction and counter-reaction with the aid of milieu changes. Only intense stimuli require central nervous and hormonal influences for regulation. Acupuncture deducts itself from this pattern – if we do not want to assume that it is capable of acting on all three mentioned levels – insofar as the various studies imply that, according to their particular morphological structure, certain points of the skin enable specific action on organs, and therefore, only activate the other regulation mechanisms secondarily, this indeed mainly denoting vegetative total readjustment after *F. Hoff*.

All studies cited mainly concern the acupuncture points or the effects achieved therewith.

Chapter IV

PULSE DIAGNOSIS

We now come to the most difficult part of the complex of energy flow regulation. The basic question – already briefly mentioned before – is as follows: How can I, in practice, determine alterations in the energy content; that is, the changes in YANG and YIN and thus the factors causing an illness, may they be general or specific to an individual organ or functional area of the various meridians? The answer is: By means of pulse diagnosis. Up to now, the reader probably tends to accept acupuncture, although it is still new to him, especially because of the information in the foregoing chapter. But now pure mysticism, or at least great subjectivity, seems to enter the picture. Before we discuss the value or worthlessness of this method of examination, allow me to describe the actual palpation procedure.

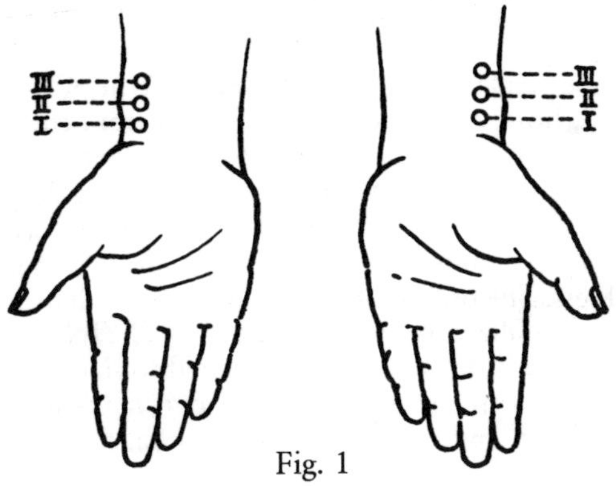

Fig. 1

The Pulse Positions: The examiner takes the pulse on both radial arteries (at the typical site) simultaneously using three fingers for each wrist. The middle finger is placed on the radial apophysis; the ring finger proximal to the apophysis next to the middle finger; the index finger distal to it. We now have three neighboring areas on which the examiner's fingers are placed. We call these areas positions. Position I is under the index finger, Position II under the middle Finger, and Position III under the ring finger. We can now differentiate the pulse beats in these three positions with the fingertips with regard to the area struck and the intensity. However, we are not only able to distinguish these three positions; we can also differentiate between right and left wrists, as well as between a deep and a superficial pulse quality. The Pulse Positions

In brief, we see the following: The examiner's three fingertips placed on the radial artery as described above are to judge the pulse quality of each individual area, on the left and on the right, and in a deep and a superficial position (identified by applying different pressures). These various qualities must also be compared to each other. All in all, we have 12 pulse positions, which correspond to the 12 meridians.

We have thus established the topographic situation. The palpating fingers should hardly move. In your first attempt at palpation, you will notice that the pulse beat felt on the middle finger is much stronger than that perceived on the other fingers. However, this is not a symptom to be evaluated, for it can be explained physiologically; the apophysis of the radius lying under the middle finger, the pulse beat there is naturally stronger. Once you have learned to mentally eliminate this difference (which only requires a little practice), you will find differences in the intensity of the pulse beat at the individual sites, especially in a patient with a disorder. This has nothing to do with pulsus celer et altus, changed blood pressure values, or various pulse frequencies with which we are familiar; such differences are of no interest to us here. The impression is much rather a tactile one in that on one occasion the pulse wave beats relatively strongly on a rather quadratic area (which corresponds to a YANG condition or abundance); another time only sweeps gently over a longer, rectangular area across the palpating fingertip and can be easily repressed or suppressed, denoting a YIN condition or emptiness. These – admittedly subjective – impressions will differ in the various positions if a disorder exists. For example, it is quite possible that a YIN meridian be found in a YANG condition and, vice versa, a YANG meridian in a YIN condition.

Taking the Pulse

Taking the Pulse: The best way to take the pulse is as follows: The patient should sit or lie opposite the examiner, who places his index, middle, and ring fingers on the radial artery bilaterally and simultaneously in the manner described above. The examiner thus establishes contact with the arterial tube with all six fingers. Then he presses down on all of them and subsequently releases the pressure only enough for the pulse beat to be just felt at all six sites. This position corresponds with the deep pulse qualitiy. In this position we find the pulse points of all YIN meridians and can now compare the specific pulse waves with each other as well as left with right.

Then, the pressure of the palpating finger is released until the pulse beat can no longer be felt on any position (without, however, removing the fingers from the surface!). The pressure is then increased only enough to allow the pulse beat to be just perceived at all sites. We now feel the superficial quality and can compare it in the same way as the deep quality. The superficial pulse always corresponds with the YANG meridians or organs and, as already mentioned, may quite frequently show YIN quality or predominately YANG quality depending on the particular underlying illness. The findings may be the same for all meridians of one group; this would correspond to a generalized disorder of the YANG-YIN equilibrium. However, the findings usually vary from position to position, from left to right, and from the superficial to the deep positions. The variations correspond to disorders in the individual organs attributed to the specific pulse positions, and thus allow a differential diagnosis to be made.

This sounds confusing indeed, but you only have to remember the following:

all YIN meridians travel along the **inner** side of the extremities and their pulse points are always in the **deep** position.

all YANG meridians travel along the **outer** side of the extremities and their pulse points are always in the **superficial** position.

With a little tactile perception ability, the practitioner will soon be able to recognize such differences. Nevertheless, the beginner usually finds too many. Therefore, I would recommend that you first practice by taking the pulse of healthy subjects, which will give you an idea of the normal range of pulse findings. Then, take the pulse of patients with obvious disorders. That will familiarize you with the specific differences. The next step is to take the pulse of all new patients who come to your office first and only afterwards take down their case history. If the history and symptoms coincide with the pulse finding, you have already taken the biggest step in learning pulse diagnosis. However, you can't expect to accomplish this in just a few weeks.

Of course, the pulse findings will not represent the precise diagnosis. The same goes for any field of medicine: one cannot draw immediate definite conclusions on the basis of one finding alone, except in very rare cases only. However, the pulse diagnosis leads us to the disturbed organ, which is often very valuable indeed, for example, in the case of an acute abdomen. An experience of my own can illustrate just how valuable and sometimes surprising this can be.

A ten-year-old boy was admitted to a children's surgical department with all the classical symptoms of an ileus both in the case history and momentary condition. In addition, his father, who accompanied him, reported that the boy had undergone an emergency operation for a volvulus at another hospital about two years prior thereto at which time he had also had the same symptoms. Purely out of habit I felt his pulse in the manner described above although this really seemed to be a clear-cut case. The pulse, however, revealed no significant change in the energetic relationships in the intestinal area, but instead, on the pulse point of the Meridian of the Spleen-Pancreas. Despite the father's protests and the scepticism of several colleagues, I cancelled the impending operation and had various tests done. A blood sugar level of 832 mg% was revealed; we had before us a very rare case of diabetic coma without loss of consciousness. After appropriate treatment, the blood sugar level dropped rapidly and the ileus symptoms disappeared. Had this boy undergone surgery, I would most probably have had to expect and be responsible for an exitus in tabula. However, had I not been familiar with pulse diagnosis, I most certainly would have operated on the basis of the apparent symptoms and the child's medical history in which no indication of diabetes could be found, not even in retrospect.

This case should awaken your interest in pulse diagnosis. After all, our predecessors – even if they lacked our present examination techniques – attributed much more significance to pulse-taking, and surely were aware of some of the differentiating signs mentioned here, albeit simply empirically. It can be argued whether it is necessary to bother with this type of examination when we should be able to achieve better and more objective results with modern diagnostic methods. However, we must not lose sight of the fact that functional disorders comprise the majority of cases in daily practice, and that these usually cannot – or at least not unequivocally – be verified with the methods of examination common today. Pulse diagnosis, however, can detect a functional disorder, thus enabling appropriate treatment – which need not necessarily be acupuncture – to be started in time. Therewith, we come one step closer to true prophylaxis, which is not always possible in medicine otherwise. Findings such as: on the upper borderline of the norm, still normal, or not yet clearly pathological, can gain considerably in informative value when combined with pulse diagnosis.

In practice, the corresponding pulse findings being available, acupuncture will be the method of choice, particularly when other diagnostic methods have failed to adequately define the cause of the disorder. Let us take cephalaea as an example, as its actual cause usually cannot be precisely determined with the usual methods of examination. Appropriate medication usually acts on the pain center or vascular supply of the cranium symptomatically only, but does not cure in the true sense of the word. Therefore, allow me to expand on the previous section on the diagnosis and treatment of headache. We often find chronic and therapy-resistant headache in the presence of pronounced disorders of the energy balance, especially of the Small Intestine, Large Intestine, and also Gallbladder meridians. If these energetic discrepancies can be adjusted, the headaches often disappear permanently, even if no local points on the head suggested by the patient's symptoms were used.

This is one reason why the points listed later on according to their indications and symptoms should not be put to repetitive stereotyped use. Of course, a physician who does not yet have a great deal of experience with the pulse diagnosis will have to start his treatments with these catalogued points. If, however, after several sessions the expected results have not yet been achieved, he must then proceed in accordance with the information acquired from the pulse. In cases like these, the change in the pulse is almost always clear enough for even the beginner to perceive.

Sources of Error in Pulse Diagnosis

Sources of Error in Pulse Diagnosis: According to the above, you might come to the conclusion that you must either study the pulse and its changes exactly and disregard the individual points' indications, or do without the pulse diagnosis and only use the points according to the list of indications. In reality, however, you should be able to do both. We must take the fact into consideration that there are people on whom the pulse cannot be taken either for anatomical or pathological reasons. These include all malformations in the wrist region, and arm amputees. In addition, no usable findings can be acquired if there is a great deal of scar tissue in the palpation area, such as from wrist slashes from attempted suicide. In cases of advanced arteriosclerosis as well, the hardened arteries will no longer be able to relay a clear finding when palpated. In everyday practice, up to 30% of pulse findings are not clearly usable. That is why you must be familiar with both methods of point selection, even if the phrase..." if not otherwise clearly indicated by the pulse" is repeatedly found in the indication lists. The pulse finding receives priority in the classical precepts handed down to us and, in fact, it and the symptoms are frequently congruent. However, if taking the pulse does not produce any clear findings – whether due to the above-mentioned abnormalities or insufficient experience on the part of the examiner – it must necessarily remain secondary to the symptomatology.

Now that we have dealt with sources of error which can be traced to the patient, let us turn to those on the part of the examiner. In the beginning, the pulses of the 2nd position are always evaluated as having YANG quality because the pulse wave is always felt stronger there than on Positions I and III. However, this is a physiological phenomenon, the radial apophysis lying under Position II. Hence, the arterial segment can yield only slightly and the pulse wave is perceived more intensely. You must first learn to compensate for this ever-present difference, that means, you must not allow all fingers to apply equal pressure, but rather, the middle fingers of each hand must apply less pressure than the other four. The best method is to establish the superficial and deep pulse qualities, as described above. You only have to watch out for the reemergence of the pulse beat under the fingertips of all six palpating fingers. We perceive the reemergence after complete suppression and subsequent release on the middle fingers of both hands first. We then maintain the pressure of the middle fingers until the pulse beat is also perceived on the other four positions and only then do we adjust evenly and simultaneously in all positions by either increasing or reducing pressure. Even though this procedure sounds so complicated, it can be mastered with a little practice.

The basic error which the beginner tends to make is feeling the pulse too long. Here, striving for the most exact comprehension of all sensations possible does not lead to progress, but rather, to the exact opposite. In the beginning, I said that pulse diagnosis is a subjective method of examination and that is why one should limit oneself to gaining a rough impression of all pulses. The first impression is always the best. The longer pressure is applied, the greater is the chance that the pulse qualities change and that the examiner is led to erroneous conclusions.

Finally, there is another problem, which I have already mentioned. It arises because in the beginning, not yet being sufficiently familiar with normal pulse variations, one tends to perceive every pulse as pathological. However, by practicing on healthy patients as I have suggested, these sources of error can be rapidly eliminated.

Nevertheless, even if you strive to avoid all these beginner's mistakes, you will often notice disorders in the energy quality not only in the one meridian which is responsible, but also in others, albeit to a lesser extent. The evaluation of these phenomena may, among other terms, be called pulse signification or pulse interpretation.

Complex Pulse Diagnosis

Complex Pulse Diagnosis: To me, this name seems to best describe the above phenomena because it means defining a complex process called forth by co-reaction of other meridians, organs, or functional groups related to the basically disturbed organ. Here, we return to the concept of partner organs which can be connected with each other via the passage points. Quite often the functional Meridian of the Triple Heater will also be irritated in the presence of a disorder in the thoracic region or abdomen. However, this simultaneous disturbance does not conform to such clear-cut laws as the rules about to be discussed, for which a diagram has been drawn (Fig. 2).

right superficial	deep		deep	left superficial
Triple Heater	Pericardium	(3rd Pos.)	Kidney	Bladder
Stomach	Spleen-Pancreas	(2nd Pos.)	Liver	Gallbladder
Large Intestine	Lung	(1st Pos.)	Heart	Small Intestine

Fig. 2 (as seen by the examiner)

The Husband-Wife Rule

The Husband-Wife Rule: We are confronted here with the flowery names handed down to us by the Chinese. However, the name of this rule makes a statement about the relationship between organs, the pulse points of which share the same position (Positions I, II, or III) and the same level (that is, superficial or deep), however, on different sides (that is, on the left or right wrist). We can also say that each of the two YANG organs in the same position are related, just as the two YIN organs of the same position are. Hence, we find the following:

Position I: Correlation between the YANG meridians Small Intestine and Large Intestine,
Position I: Correlation between the YIN meridians Heart and Lung,
Position II: Correlation between the YANG meridians Gallbladder and Stomach,
Position II: Correlation between the YIN meridians Liver and Spleen-Pancreas,
Position III: Correlation between the YANG meridians Bladder and Triple Heater,
Position III: Correlation between the YIN meridians Kidney and Pericardium (Envelope of the Heart).

I do not wish to confuse you at this point by using this rule to create energetic equilibrium. For the moment, I just want to draw your attention to the possibility of there being a disorder in both meridians related as above. These connections seem functionally and anatomically both correct and plausible also from our medical perspectives. If, for example, there is a disorder in the Gallbladder Meridian, such as in cholecystitis, it is absolutely feasible that a simultaneous disturbance in the Stomach Meridian will be found.

The Mother-Son Rule

The Mother-Son Rule: This rule is based on the sequence of the meridians in the circulation of energy. In keeping therewith, the meridian preceding an organ is called its mother and the meridian following it is called its son. It follows that the mother is always willing to give energy, while the son is willing to receive it. For example, if we want to tonify the Heart Meridian in particular, we can also tonify its mother (the Meridian of the Spleen-Pancreas in the circulation of energy). This will achieve a greater influx of YANG energy. On the other hand, if we want to sedate the Heart Meridian to a large extent, we acupuncture its sedation point (with a silver needle) and the sedation point of its son (the Small Intestine).

In the latter case, however, we are also dealing with partner organs. That is not the case in the first example. When partner meridians are involved, we can also use the passage point, and thus, less needles. This example shows us that different rules can sometimes overlap. This should not be seen as a disadvantage, but rather, it gives us even more ways of regulating energy. The ability to diagnose the pulse is necessary for applying these rules via the above pairs. The mother-son rule surpasses the concept of partner organs and takes the sequence of the circulation of energy into consideration, the regulation of energy being carried out via the respective sedation or tonification points of both meridians. If we happen to be dealing with partner organs, which are in opposite energetic conditions at the outset, we can use the passage point instead of the previously-mentioned main points.

The Midday-Midnight Rule

The Midday-Midnight Rule: In regard to this rule, please recall the so-called maximum times, as presented in the table listing the sequence of the meridians. The Chinese hour corresponds to two hours of our time. Each organ is given a double hour, thus the 12 meridians cover a 24-hour period. Two organs are always in opposition night and day, for example Heart (12:00 noon – 2:00 PM) and Gallbladder (12:00 midnight – 2:00 AM). That is, one YANG and one YIN organ always stand in opposition to each other. If the Heart Meridian is tonified during its maximum time via its tonification point with a gold needle, a sedation of the opposing YANG Meridian of the Gallbladder will be achieved, and vice-versa (Fig. 3).

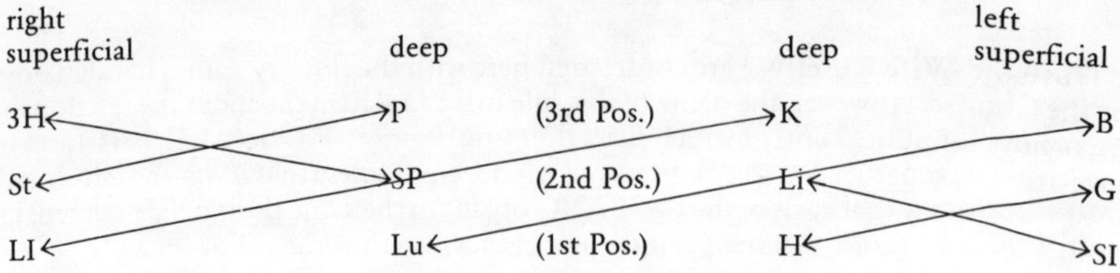

Fig. 3 (as seen by the examiner)

All that has been said up to now is certainly very confusing. Let me point out the fact that you will seldom have to employ all the possibilities described at the same time. On the other hand, these rules will often prove to be valuable when used alone.

Diagnostic Synthesis of the Three Rules

Diagnostic Synthesis of the Three Rules: We shall now attempt to establish a type of synthesis. If acupuncture really is a comprehensive method of healing unto itself, then all of these rules must not only be reflected in the regulation of the pulse, but also in the symptomatology regarding the indicated points. This could then be particularly helpful to the physician who has little experience with pulse diagnosis, as he could in the beginning apply the symptomatology of the points and would subsequently recognize the time-saving effect of pulse-taking and the information obtained therefrom.

Let's take the following case as an example. The Meridian of the Small Intestine is in a YANG condition. We have said that the Meridian of the Small Intestine's influence goes above and beyond its own organ, especially spasmolytically, and has a general harmonizing action on all mucous membranes. According to the above rules, the Meridian of the Small Intestine is related

a) to the Meridian of the Heart via the passage point SI 7,
b) to the Meridian of the Bladder according to the mother-son rule. As the Small Intestine is in a YANG condition in our example, we must also sedate the son (the Meridian of the Bladder) with the sedation point of the Bladder, B 65.
c) to the Meridian of the Large Intestine according to the husband-wife rule. As the meridians oppose each other according to this rule, the Large Intestine must be tonified is the Small Intestine is to be sedated in this case, using its tonification point, LI 11,
d) to the Meridian of the Liver according to the midday-midnight rule. Here too, we are confronted with an opposition such as in the husband-wife rule. Therefore, we must also tonify the Meridian of the Liver via its tonification point, Li 9.

We have found all these points by means of pulse diagnosis. The meridians mentioned in the above compilation will also reveal themselves in the same pulse quality even in more difficult cases. Thus, the Small Intestine and Bladder Meridians will be found to be in a YANG state; the Large Intestine and Liver Meridians in a YIN state. If the Meridian of the Heart is also in a YIN state, we can use the passage point, SI 7; in doing so, we achieve an internal energy balance between the Heart and Small Intestine Meridians. However, should the Meridian of the Heart also be in a YANG state, the passage point cannot be used.

Let us look at the above-mentioned points and meridians with reference to their indications or symptoms and how they relate. In keeping with the above list we begin with

a) SI 7, passage point to the Meridian of the Heart (partner organ).
Indications: Pain in the arm, eye inflammations.
b) B 65, sedation point of the Bladder, used acccording to the mother-son rule.
Indications: Cervical syndrome with radiating pain, eye inflammations.
c) LI 11, tonification point of the Large Intestine, used according to the husband-wife rule.
Indications: General spasm, pain in the shoulder and arm, constipation.
d) LI 9, tonification point of the Liver, used according to the midday-midnight rule.
Indications: General spasm, migrating pain, constipation.

If we now compare the most important point that we have discovered on the basis of pulse diagnosis, that is, the sedation point of the Meridian of the Small Intestine, it revealing the greatest disturbance and a YANG state, hence, SI 8, we see its indications being: general spasm, pain in the shoulder and arm, and constipation. Hence, absolute congruity with LI 11 regarding the symptoms or indications, and a partial correspondence to the other mentioned points as well as between these themselves.

Therapeutic Synthesis of the Three Rules

Therapeutic Synthesis of the Three Rules: If we obtain a pulse finding which leads us to the above rules and points, then the patient too will almost always describe the above-mentioned symptoms. Should we not yet be able to select the above points on the basis of the pulse, we can also identify and use the same points according to the list of symptoms and knowledge of the three rules, however, this is more time-consuming. By inserting the appropriate gold or silver needles in all points, we will quickly achieve a balance of energy, and as a result, the complaints will also disappear. However, if the patient complains of only one or two of the above symptoms, we use the points corresponding thereto. The body practically chooses the appropriate reaction itself and deals with the complaints. The entire process is like that of a computer.

Having summarized the most important basics of acupuncture, we receive the impression that the precepts of acupuncture form an incredibly compact unity. It is a complex system with no gaps, and with the widest scope of use imaginable. The inherent combination possibilities are vast. To avoid confusion and to establish changes in the pulse findings, I suggest taking down exact records. The best method is to use the above diagram because it provides a general view of the possible connections between the meridians and the energetic conditions may be recorded at the same time. Using the simplest method, we record a YANG condition with a plus sign and a YIN condition with a minus sign. In doing so, we also signify all YANG states as conditions of abundance, and all YIN states as conditions of deficit. If the pulse beat on the fingertip on one of the positions is extremely strong, we can record it with three plus signs. If it is very strong, we use two plus signs; if it is strong, one. Vice-versa, we record a weak beat with one to three minus signs. Of course, this way of measuring is always subjective and individual, but because its consequences remain practically constant in all cases, it is unobtrusive and practical.

One thing is important: In case of doubt, the beginner should not refer to an uncertain pulse finding for diagnosis and therapy, but rather revert to the points' symptomatology. In such cases, we are often confronted with a complex picture, that is, the dominating disturbance masks another, usually more profound, disorder. After the first few treatments, a significant change in the pulse finding of such cases is found, and treatment must then be adjusted accordingly. The same applies when treatment is symptomatic. For the latter, the records suggested above are especially useful. However, it is necessary in cases like these – or better yet, in all cases – to inform the patient prior to therapy, because a treatment which often appears to be short and simple at first frequently unveils other conditions which require further treatment. This is indirect proof that acupuncture is a therapy having a strong influence on regulation.

In summarizing, we can say that pulse diagnosis provides us with fast information about the patient. With this information we can immediately initiate therapy purely to balance energy, and as a result, we will see many complaints disappear. However, it may happen that the complaints which bring the patient to the physician in the first place prove to be superimposed on one or more other general disorders. If the pulse finding is unclear, one should proceed according to the symptoms; this applies especially to the beginner. The various laws have revealed great correlations. These are reflected in the symptomatology and can also be applied when treatment is not to be based on the pulse diagnosis.

Chapter V

THE TECHNIQUE OF ACUPUNCTURE AND THE REACTIONS IT CAUSES

Up to this point, the energy, its paths of conduction (the meridians), and its switching locations (the points) have been discussed in detail, as have the ways of establishing energetic changes, and the rules for controlling them. Now, let us delve into the actual technique of acupuncture. The word acupuncture is a Latin technical term consisting of acus – needle, and punctura – puncture. The most obvious process in this therapy, the needling of points on the skin, was taken as name. However, in reality, needling is the consequence of all or many of the considerations we have discussed. It is the agent which utilizes all these concepts and shall now be described in more detail.

The Technique of Needling

The Technique of Needling: Appropriate points are selected on the basis of the pulse diagnosis and/or evaluation of the symptoms, and needled with gold, silver, or steel needles. In general, these needles are inserted 2-8 mm into the skin, depending on the part of the body being needled, and as close the point's center as possible. Should the needle miss the point's center, peripheral needling in the same direction as the meridian's course (that is, an upward or downward deviation) will reduce the effect to a lesser degree than would lateral or medial deviation from the point's center. As we have already seen, a combination of several points is usually used. In the following list of symptoms, only the abbreviated names of the points are given, whereby it must be again stressed that for each of these points, you must count 2 needles (one on the left and one on the right side of the body), and therefore, the number of needles is usually twofold that of the points. Only the so-called vessels (TOU-MO and JENN-MO) are exceptions. You should always try to use 14 needles or less per session. The needles are inserted one after the other, quickly and with a slight rotation to keep the pain caused by penetrating the skin at a minimum. We usually insert gold needles first because they stay in the tissue longer. The needles are left in place for 5-10 minutes on the average whereby extensions or reductions of this period are possible. Thereafter, distinct red halos appear around the inserted needles, which some authors consider to be the result of histamine release. On taut skin areas, such as the back of the hand, etc., the red halos are considerably less pronounced, usually hardly noticeable. There is a simple method of determining when the needles have been in the tissue long enough. The inserted needle can of course be removed at any time. However, if we pull very carefully on a needle which has just been inserted, we will see that the skin immediately protrudes around the site of insertion, and the needle can only be removed with some effort. However, if we wait 5 or 10 minutes without touching the needle, and then just slightly pull on it, it easily slips out of the skin. Of course, pulling on the needle after insertion is for demonstration purposes only; as a rule, it is not touched. Only when the above-described red halos have appeared around the needle do we remove it. If this cannot be easily ascertained, for example, on certain body areas, we pull lightly on the needle to test whether the skin still protrudes around it. If not, and the needle slides out easily, the session may be considered over. The redness disappears within a few minutes after the needle has been removed. Even if the needles have been inserted correctly, there may be rare instances of slight bleeding, or excretion of a few drops of blood from the point. Simple compression is quite sufficient, so there should be no hematoma.

Depending on the body area to be needled, the needle is inserted either perpendicularly or at an approx. angle of about 60°. According to the depth of insertion, the needles either remain upright in the tissue or they tilt immediately. After some time, almost all the needles tilt while still in the skin. This is a signal that the session is nearly over. After the needle has been inserted, the patient often describes a feeling of warmth or a sensation similar to that when a weak source of electricity is touched; sometimes a sort of tingling. Usually, these sensations are not limited to the site of needle insertion only, but rather radiate along part of the meridian, usually, however, independent of the direction of the energy's course.

Special Needling Techniques

Special Needling Techniques: Quite often, especially for all types of paralysis, severe pain, etc., the needles are inserted deeper than described above. In the Far East in particular, needles are generally inserted deeper than in the West. Personally, I am not in favor of inserting the needle too deeply. Perhaps somewhat more time is required to achieve desired results when the needle is inserted superficially, but results are achieved just the same without the risk of injury. However, when the needle is inserted deeper, a hot sensation, like a weak electric shock, travels a considerable distance along the meridian. This phenomenon can be prognostically evaluated as favorable in cases of paralysis, muscular dystrophy, etc. This technique is also used for diagnostic purposes in cases of paralysis. Even if this phenomenon appears on only one of the so-called paralysis points during test treatment, there is hope for the patient, and the use of acupunctural therapy is justified. Deep insertion of the needle usually eliminates the criterion of the skin bulging around the needle. So you have to watch the clock, whereby other factors must also be taken into consideration. For example, if the patient feels cold, the session will take significantly longer than on a warm or even humid summer day. The needles stay in the skin of very nervous, frightened, or very sensitive patients for a considerably shorter period of time than in that of phlegmatic patients. Occasionally, the needle may have to be removed again immediately after it has been inserted.

The Ou-Rou Method

The Ou-Rou Method: This is a very special technique. It is used for inflammations of the small finger joints or for vascular disorders in the hand and fingers only. Here, a normal acupuncture needle is inserted and immediately removed at each end of the interphalangeal skin fold which is formed when the finger is bent, in other words, the skin is just pricked. In contrast to the other types of needling, even deep insertion, this form of treatment is quite painful. It is performed on all affected fingers and is astonishingly successful for the above indications, its use thus being justified. Six locations are pricked on each finger; only four on the thumb of course. For vascular disorders of the hands and fingers in this method, one silver needle is inserted at the vola manus between the head of each of the distal metacarpal bones. These needles are left in the tissue until the originally livid color of the fingers is replaced by a distinct, healthy rosiness. At the same time, the red halo, appearing around the inserted needle at the beginning as usual, turns white, and a distinct sensation of warmth is felt both by the patient as well as by the physician. Nevertheless, these points are relatively painful.

Normally, the insertion of the needles is only slightly painful, especially the first few times. However, it becomes increasingly more painful as the condition treated improves, which can be evaluated diagnostically as well as prognostically, although a true pain gauge can never be achieved. If the patient finds insertion of the needles intolerable, he is either a hypochondriac or has psychopathic tendencies.

The "Permanent" or Fastened Needle

The "Permanent" or Fastened Needle: This is the opposite of the Ou-Rou method just described. Here, special needles which look like thumbtacks with a pin guide are employed. They are used especially for recurrent, short spasms, such as tics. They are inserted in the appropriate points and held in place with two crossed adhesive strips. Hence, they remain in place for several hours or even days. In contrast to the other, common needling techniques, this can sometimes cause minor local infection. Therefore, the patient must be examined daily or made aware of the danger of secondary infection. If an infection develops, the needle must be removed immediately and only replaced one week after the infection has healed up at the earliest. This technique is rarely used; I have only mentioned it for the sake of completeness.

The Various Types of Needles

The Various Types of Needles: The beginning acupuncturist's kit should contain the following:

2 gold facial needles
2 silver facial needles
2 large gold needles
4 small gold needles
4 large silver needles
6 small silver needles
2 Japanese needles with a guide tube (silver or steel).

As the name implies, facial needles are used mainly for points on the face or on tender areas of the skin. These thin needles are used because these areas are more sensitive. They should only be used for these areas, as otherwise they might easily bend or even break. Large and small needles on the other hand differ in length only; their diameter is just about the same. They are selected mainly according to how much fatty tissue there is on the point to be needled. All needles have a pin guide with which they are held by the physician and inserted using slight rotation as close to the center of the point as possible. The deeper the point lies, e.g. in isolated spasms from athletic injuries, or protective spasm as a result of rheumatic illnesses, the more difficult locating the center of the point becomes. The so-called Japanese needles are helpful in such cases. These are usually made of silver or steel and the needle itself is somewhat longer than the tube around it. When inserting the needle, the guide tube is aimed so that the needle is directed exactly at the deep spasm. Then, the protruding end of the inserted Japanese needle is pushed with the finger, or later, with another needle, until the cramped spot is reached or the direction of the inserted needle can no longer be changed. The tube around the Japanese needle can then be pulled off. These needles are thinner than the common gold or silver needles, and thus, much more flexible. Therefore, when they are inserted deeper, as is required for the above indications, paralyses, etc., they may yield and miss their target. The guide tube is used to avoid this. The Japanese needles can also be used to produce micro-bleeding, as is sometimes required especially at the so-called metabolic points in skin diseases. However, there are already special needles for this on the market which have a hooked tip and thus cause local bleeding in any case. An example of such a point is Bladder 54 in the middle of the popliteal space. As already mentioned, needling usually causes no bleeding whatsoever; occasionally, bleeding can be due to an aberration of the course of a vessel. Bleeding of this type, like that purposely caused, ceases immediately upon slight compression and may leave a small bruise at the most.

To recapitulate, fastened or "permanent" needles look like thumbtacks with a small pin guide. They are not essential for the beginner. Finally, there are moxa needles. These are normal acupuncture needles made out of various metals, having a little cup on the top instead of a guide, in which moxa (dried artemesia weed) is burned, thus heating the needle. This method too is rarely used and is not essential for the beginner.

Comparison of the Effects of Gold and Silver Needles

Comparison of the Effects of Gold and Silver Needles: Some of the questions most frequently asked in acupuncture are, "What is the difference between gold and silver needles?" And, "When should which be used?" "Is there a difference in the effect?" "Is there proof thereof?" Again, the simplest answer is found in the old traditional precepts. Tonifying characteristics are attributed to the gold needle (yellow metal) and sedative effects to the silver (white metal). This rule of thumb has proved useful in practice. However, scientific proof is a more complicated matter. In my opinion, despite many studies, there is no final proof as of yet. For example, *Te Suck Song,* Korea, found variations in the 17 α-ketosterone of 24-hour urine depending on the metal used. To me, these studies do not seem to be particularly significant and are also not reliable because of the small number of patients investigated. *Fujita* and *Minami* from Japan also studied this problem. Artificial indurations were produced through massage of the shoulder area of previously albumin-sensitized rabbits. The rabbits were subsequently divided into three groups, the first receiving no subsequent therapy; the second being needled unilaterally with silver needles (theoretically correct metal), and the third group with gold needles, again unilaterally (the wrong metal). Changes in the indurations were scrutinized both by palpation and histologically. Clear differences were revealed. The greatest difference existed between the untreated and treated groups. In the latter two, there was a reduction in size and softening of the indurations; in the untreated animals, changes of this type were hardly perceptible.

However, histologically, the untreated group and the group treated with gold needles were similar. The group which had been treated with silver needles differed distinctly. Thus, the authors arrived at the conclusion that there must be a difference between gold and silver needles and consider the choice of metal important in the treatment of allergies.

Nakatani considers the difference slight and negligible. *Prinzing* considers the difference significant on the basis of urograms and pharmacological tests. *Manaka,* who studied the different actions of varying points, had a diverging approach. He was able to establish a difference in effect especially when the sedation or tonification point was used.

Prodescu demonstrates other contrasts: He studied the change in the production of bile in dogs in a double experiment. First, he used silver needles, and after a suitable interval, gold needles. The results obtained were then compared with the results after the administration of Decholin® (acidum dehydrocholicum). Needle therapy achieved more pronounced effects than did Decholin®. At first, the difference between gold and silver needles did not seem noteworthy, however, after-treatment revealed gold needles as having a more favorable effect than silver.

Wogralik measured the electric potential of the different needles. With the gold needles commonly used, he was able to establish a potential of +0.285; with silver needles, a potential of +0.048 according to the hydrogen scale. That means that there is a distinct difference between these two metals. This difference gains significance when its relationship to the surrounding tissue is examined, because here, the silver needle can even be proved negative in comparison to tissue.

We must not allow ourselves to be confused by these diverging opinions. We know that the potential of tissue is changed in any case by insertion of the needle, and we can use the potential gradient produced by these two different metals for therapeutic purposes. Therefore, we should adhere to the old rule that needles of both metals should be used in each acupuncture session, however, not in a 1 to 1 relationship, but rather always 3 to 4 times as many silver needles as gold needles. Experience has taught us that silver has a sedating action psychologically as well as in regard to the reduction of inflammation, particularly in nonspecific inflammatory conditions, these constituting a large number of cases indicated for acupuncture treatment.

Nevertheless, the selection of the correct points seems to be more important than the difference between metals. After all, with the right points, similar effects can also be achieved with steel needles, or even point massage. Last but not least, if we still prefer to use precious metals, the oligodynamic effect thereof is a good reason for doing so. Therefore, when using precious metals for acupuncture, infections need hardly be feared, because the needles are not hollow, but solid. However, it should be stressed that today, if for no other than forensic reasons, all needles must be sterilized. This causes rapid discoloration of silver needles, less so of gold, which is why we suggest sterilizing precious metal needles in an autoclave only.

Before actual insertion, they should be cleansed with a wad of cotton soaked with a disinfectant, such as Merfen Tincture® (Zyma Pharmaceutical Company, Switzerland). In other words, the needles to be used are taken from their container and placed in the left hand in the wad of cotton soaked with, for example, Merfen tincture. Each needle is pulled through the wad before being inserted into the skin. I sterilize my needles in a hot air sterilizer or autoclave. It goes without saying that steel needles have no oligodynamic effect and must always be sterilized before use. The procedure is the same for fastened or "permanent" needles. If you have a larger number of patients, having several sets of needles is advisable, thus avoiding time-consuming interruption for sterilization. There are also containers on the market which are designed to hold a larger number of needles, including Japanese needles. The needles hang in these containers, so that the tips are not damaged. Blunt needles can be sharpened several times on an oilstone. This procedure helps a few times, but ultimately, the needle must be replaced. The needles should be counted before and after every treatment, as some may fall out and slip into the patient's clothing.

In summarizing the different effects of gold and silver needles, we can say that though a difference has not yet been scientifically proven, not only experience and the laws of the regulation of energy require the use of these needles, but, the potential gradient between them and the tissue, as well as their oligodynamic effect can only be of advantage.

Complications During an Acupuncture Treatment

Complications During an Acupuncture Treatment: Let me begin by saying that no serious complications arise in acupuncture. Nevertheless, there are sometimes difficulties which should be discussed at this point. The most frequent is the patient's fear of the first needle. There are several ways of combatting this. First, you must make the patient aware of the fact that it will indeed be a little painful. Other patients have probably told him so already, but they usually tend to either underplay or exaggerate. Before the first needle is inserted, palpate the skin area which is to be needled to check for tension. If you have the impression that the patient is tense because he is afraid, massage each point with the fingertip before inserting the needle. The Chinese recommend a light, circular motion counterclockwise on the point to calm, as is done in Chinese massage. This quickly relaxes the tense skin area, and the needle can then be inserted easily to the required depth with a slight rotation. You can determine this depth by spreading one finger of the guiding hand out so that it strikes the skin when the depth has been reached and thus acts as a brake. However, a single motion will not suffice for deeper needle insertion. The latter requires that, the cutis having been penetrated, you continue to insert the needle deeper by lightly rotating it until the above-described "shock" has been released. Then, immediately release pressure and leave the needle in place.

Here, too, rotating the needle into the skin is considered important. Consistent with the precepts of Chinese massage, a tonifying action is attributed to clockwise rotation of the needle, and a sedating action to counterclockwise rotation. Thus, when the needles are inserted, you must take the characteristics of each point into consideration, and choose the direction in which the needle should be rotated accordingly.

It the patient is particularly anxious or sensitive, I recommend having him cough while the needle is being inserted. After the point has been exactly located, I tell the patient to cough. At the height of the cough impetus, extensive relaxation takes place, and the needle slides quickly and unnoticed to the desired depth, which, again, can be controlled by propping a finger against the skin.

Though rare, it can happen that a patient collapses; the cause is usually psychological. These patients are almost always males, and robust persons at that. I have never experienced a woman collapsing. Therefore, it is recommended that such patients always receive treatment lying down. Basically, every new patient should be treated lying down the first few times. Later, he or she can be treated while sitting, or even standing if necessary. If the patient collapses despite this precaution, acupuncture is also the quickest and best remedy. The points H 9 and P 9 are used. H 9 is found 2 mm proximal and medial to the radial corner of the cuticle of the small finger; P 9 on the middle finger in the same position. Both are tonification points of their respective meridians and can be acupunctured with a gold needle. By the way, the above applies to cases of collapse in general, and not only to those due to acupuncture. Usually, needling is not even necessary; strong pressure with the fingernail on these points is sufficient. This too stems from the precepts of Chinese massage, and the practical applications can be summarized as follows: To tonify, either apply strong pressure to the point with your fingernail or massage it in a clockwise circular motion. To sedate, massage the point with the fingertip using slight pressure in a counterclockwise circular motion. With this method, you can even avoid using needles on children sometimes – less frequently on adults – and achieve similar results.

When Needles Fall Out Prematurely

When Needles Fall Out Prematurely: This phenomenon is seen quite often. The needles usually drop out sooner than expected as a result of cramping caused by psychological tension. Sometimes this is due to purely physical reasons, e.g. if the patient has had to remain motionless in an uncomfortable position. Therefore, if needles have been inserted in the head, the patient should avoid talking during the first phase, as the resulting movements of the facial muscles can cause the needles to sway and fall out. Needles which have fallen out should be reinserted. However, the needle should not be reinserted in the same point more than twice during one session. Of course, the reaction may be faster at one point than at others. This is the case when the reinserted needle falls out again after a matter of seconds, or if the red halo is very pronounced. In that case, do not reinsert the needle, but rather wait until a distinct reaction has appeared on all the other points. Of course, the above does not apply to a needle which has been inserted too superficially as the beginning acupuncturist tends to do.

Abnormalities and After-Bleeding

Abnormalities and After-Bleeding: Occasionally, a point is located within a skin structure (warts, pigmentation etc.). Naturally, you should not insert the needle into these points, especially where there are pigmented warts. Furthermore, ulcers of the leg usually cover the area of the point especially suitable for treatment thereof (SP 6). In such cases, you must select other points (according to symptomatology or the rules of the regulation of energy) which are not covered by defects of this type. Substitutes can always be found.

Scars over points or meridians are a different matter. Histological research has shown that connective tissue usually replaces the destroyed specific tissue. That means that the original function cannot be reinstated; new connective tissue can only act supportively to promote the function of the remaining specific tissue. It is capable of this as it intervenes in the primitive regulative action of the interstice, as we have discussed earlier. However, this is only possible if the formation of substitute tissue is not disturbed. Otherwise, a locus of irritation (nowadays, a more suitable term would be focus) is formed, and around it, a field of irritation. Both are able to change the environment and the energetic process in this area, usually to a disadvantage.

Therefore, it may happen that patients with scars altered in the above sense seem to be blocked off from the points and meridians lying on those areas, that is, the applied stimulus cannot break through. Quite often, the ability to react can be reinstated in such cases by inserting several silver needles around the scar or by injecting novocain or impletol, etc. In all cases of abnormal reactions to acupuncture, and where there appear to be discrepancies in the case history, scars of this kind, which need not be very large and which usually look completely normal on the surface, must be taken into consideration. Such scars can be recognized as loci or fields of irritation on the basis of electrical resistance measurement values obtained with the previously described point detectors.

Finally, an aberrant vessel can also traverse a point. If it is visible, avoid inserting the needle into it or select the angle of insertion accordingly to avoid bleeding. The same applies to bruises which have appeared during or after the previous treatment. Bleeding immediately after removal of the needles can always be stopped by simple compression, and requires no further treatment. Once in a great while, clothing may rub, or the patient himself scratches the treated location causing secondary infections. These are treated locally accordingly.

Edema of the joints or of the lower legs is not a contra-indication for using a point in that area. After the treatment, secretion of parenchymatous fluid is observed, which may continue for some time. In such cases, a sterile gauze strip should be applied.

Hypersensitive reactions, especially to silver, are extremely rare. Nevertheless, in such cases, steel needles should be tried.

In summarizing, we can say that during and immediately after an acupuncture treatment, complications may arise, which, however, rarely lead to serious incidents. The suitable counter-measures have been mentioned, and we have also noted the problems sometimes arising due to scar tissue alterations.

Post-Acupuncture Reactions

Post-Acupuncture Reactions: I have already discussed the needles and the technique of inserting them (without yet going into details on the direction in which the needle is to be inserted, that is, in the same or opposite direction of the flow of energy, or the synchronization of needle insertion with the patient's breathing), as well as the length of time the needles are left in place, and various possible complications. Now, we must talk about the reactions to the treatment and the intervals between each session. I have already mentioned the initial reactions: the red halos around the inserted needle, and, should they not be distinct, the phenomenon of the skin no longer protruding when the needle is ready to be removed. I have also mentioned that the length of time before these phenomena appear may vary greatly and depends on the patient's constitution, momentary condition, the temperature outside and in the treatment room; hence, on endogenous as well as exogenous factors.

If there is no reaction at all to a correctly selected and executed treatment, you must consider the possibility of unresponsiveness. I have already mentioned the four normal curves in the section on vegetative regulation. There, we noted that unresponsiveness renders an acupuncture treatment futile. We may be faced with total or partial unresponsiveness. The Elpimed® (extract from specifically treated blood) insulin alternating therapy is sometimes able to combat total unresponsiveness: Elpimed® (after data from *Lutz* and *Pischinger)* is administered three times within a few days, this promoting basic reactions. After three days, this therapy is interrupted and a single dose of 10 to 15 units unmodified insulin, the antagonist of Elpimed® is given. After repeating this cycle several times as a rule, such cases are usually seen to respond, and acupuncture may be applied accordingly.

In cases of partial unresponsiveness, you may observe a general reaction, but the desired specific reaction is not achieved. This condition is usually caused by fields of disturbance, which must be eliminated first. Usually, these fields of disturbance (foci) reveal themselves by suddenly becoming acute within the first four sessions. These processes are usually so intense that surgical elimination of the foci is the only solution. After a recuperation phase of about three weeks, the body is able to react positively and rapidly to acupuncture therapy.

The Intervals between Treatments

The Intervals between Treatments: This aspect is closely related to the reaction types. The 4 different types after *Pischinger* are revealed analogously in practice. The interval length between treatments depends wholly thereupon. The patient whose response corresponds to the normal curve usually reacts with a short-term initial improvement, this at times even resembling the "Sekundenphänomen" after *Huneke* (disappearance of pain within seconds). However, this phase usually only lasts for a matter of hours, or a few days at the most, then the status quo ante returns. After the second – more often after the third – treatment, this type of patient reacts with distinct exacerbation. These exacerbations can be considered reactive not only because they correspond to the comparative curves, but also because of the fact that otherwise effective pain-killing drugs are ineffectual during this phase. After this phase, however, the drugs may again be used effectively if necessary, even if the complaints or pain are of the same intensity. A basic change in the reaction begins to take place after the fourth treatment, characterized by a reduction in the complaints. Further treatments, which can range from 6-12 depending on the individual, are then necessary. Deviations from these guidelines are not infrequent, therefore, don't give up too soon. The results achieved in this group are usually long-lasting. The reactions as such are worsening of complaints, these often becoming more intense than prior to treatment, thus indicating a more extensive disorder than was to be expected on the basis of the patient's descriptions. This is comparable to reactions to spa therapy (which, after all, also stimulates the skin).

Another important fact is that reactions of this type do not only persist throughout the entire treatment as such, but also reveal themselves after each individual session, albeit to a lesser extent. Therefore, we are faced with two superimposed curves, which are similar in their general courses, but completely different temporally. We also find this superimposition in the other reaction types corresponding to the other standard curves. After the normal reaction curve, with which we have now become familiar, comes the second most common form, which is more pleasant for the patient.

This second group shows a striking improvement already after the first treatment; sometimes a second treatment is no longer even necessary, as the complaints have disappeared. In these cases, as well as in all patients with acute processes, these comprising the minority of patients seeking acupuncture treatment, further treatment should be postponed when there has been a spectacular improvement of this kind. Otherwise, the effect so easily acquired can be extinguished. Acupuncture is a harmonizing therapy, and cannot achieve results which surpass the norm. Therefore, we cannot turn good into excellent if the body does not already have the capacity to do so itself, this having been demonstrated in the past, even if only temporarily. If you nevertheless elect to continue treatment on such patients, you will destroy the normal regulation already achieved and you will then have to begin anew on a much more profound basis. Let this be an urgent warning against attempting "prophylaxis" otherwise not uncommon in medicine for this reaction group. Because of the fact that the various reaction types cannot be distinguished in advance, use the above-described, typical processes as guidelines.

As pleasant for the patient and spectacular for one's reputation this second group seems to be, the achieved effects do not last nearly as long as those achieved in the first group. Usually, these patients return after a year with the same or similar complaints, which, however, again disappear just as rapidly after acupuncture treatment.

To a certain extent, similar effects can be observed in the so-called long-term treatment cases *(Bischko)*. The difference is that in cases of long-term treatment, the reversibility of the condition is only limited or the patient has a limited resistance and response capacity. In contrast to the second group, true improvement cannot be achieved, but rather, the complaints only appear to improve. However, if treatment is discontinued for a longer period of time, external influences extinguish the effect and it can only be reinstated again with some effort. Thus, in long-term treatment cases, there is no real improvement, but rather, the body adapts to the specific disorder. Most long-term treatment patients require more frequent treatments, intervals between individual sessions lasting a few months at the most; often only a few weeks. Long-term treatment of this type is relatively rare; results can only be determined from a negative standpoint: When the patient doesn't come for treatment, he feels worse; when he comes, he feels better – in other words, a type of substitution therapy.

Finally, we come to the third group. In these cases, the first treatment results in worsening of the condition, which slowly improves after further treatments (but does at times continue to get worse). These cases require a great deal of patience on the part of the patient as well as the physician, and a longer treatment period. The contrast to the non-responder is clearly seen by the presence of reactions, albeit negative ones. Due to the considerable individual variations in such patients, there are no guidelines as to how long treatment will be required. This is without doubt the most unpleasant response form for both patient and physician.

Thus, the above shows how important it is that the patient cooperates and observes his own reactions to acupuncture. This, however, is problematic, as most people have forgotten how to observe and therefore cannot provide useful data. Some go to the opposite extreme which, being basically iatrogenic, must be combatted. Thus, we receive either too much or too little information from the patient. Therefore, you must literally teach the patient to observe himself correctly. You can usually obtain a good picture of the patient's personality with a few indirect, but not leading, questions. Maintaining good contact with the physician who referred the patient and having him perform occasional check-ups have proven valuable.

You will learn to reliably differentiate these four principal types faster than you might expect at this point. The normal group comprises about 75% of all cases; the positive reaction group, about 15%. The remainder is divided fairly evenly between patients having negative reactions and those who are non-responders.

As already mentioned, weather conditions must also be taken into consideration when evaluating the reactions. The phenomena of inversion and sudden changes in humidity described by *Maresch* may throw a completely different light on the in fact good observations a patient has made. In areas where no continual recordings of such meteorological aspects are made, informative conclusions may easily be drawn on the basis of the changes one feels oneself compared to those reported by patients who are sensitive to weather changes. With experience, and with a large number of patients, this should present no problem.

Typical Treatment Intervals

Typical Treatment Intervals: We may assume that the best length for the interval between individual sessions is 5-7 days. Therefore, intervals of one week are the most practical for a normal office. Cases of paralysis are a different matter, daily treatments over a certain period being common. Why does an interval of one week seem correct? According to studies by *Kellner* (quoted in lectures by *Bischko* and *Feucht),* acupuncture produces a microwound which is also subject to the laws of wound healing. Here, we mainly differentiate two phases: a beginning regression and then subsequent repair. The regression consists of several rapid processes aimed at maintaining the remaining vital tissue, and demarcation of tissue which is becoming necrotic. In wound healing, we distinguish an initial fermentation phase which proceeds parallel to demarcation. This demarcation is achieved by the infiltration of granulocytes and leucocytes. Thereafter, phagocytic, mononuclear cells appear, which survive the two preceding phases. After 36 hours, acid mucopolysaccharides may be detected and observed up to the third day. Only on the fifth or sixth day, upon the release of water withheld prior thereto to achieve substratum transport, have the conditions required for actual repair been created. This is the second great phase of wound healing.

Wound healing can be interrupted in any of its phases, whereby the disturbance will vary depending on the momentary phase of wound healing. An area thus disturbed can develop into a focus and center of greater, irritating, energetic processes. Therefore, maintain intervals of one week whenever possible. Occasionally, it may be necessary to perform several treatments within a short period of time on, for example, patients from other cities or countries, performing artists, etc., thus reducing the normal intervals between treatments. However, I wish to stress that a concentrated treatment series may call forth intensified reactions, these usually being of a negative nature.

Atypical Treatment Intervals

Atypical Treatment Intervals: As a rule, all these cases clearly show that the individual treatments, performed at intervals of only two or three days, accumulate, because during the period following the first reaction, a second, or even third, reaction is superposed. The period of blockage to a new stimulus is over after about 20 to 30 minutes, however, the reaction persists for several days, as mentioned in the section on wound healing. Thus, in all of these cases, we usually see intense exacerbation (similar to the negative reaction phase discussed previously), which may persist after the treatment has been ended. Therefore, before you give an intensive treatment series of this type, you must warn the patient that the concentration of stimuli may cause his condition to worsen. Indeed, he may even feel worse than prior to treatment. There should be a pause of one to two months following concentrated treatment of this type. The effect thereof can only be determined after this period of time has elapsed. Desired results will be achieved if the disorder was recognized and dealt with correctly right from the beginning. It is very difficult to make corrections or changes in the therapy program when treatment is administered that frequently. Particularly the beginner will find this extremely problematic.

Treatment at intervals which are longer than one week, again due to external influences, are a different matter. Of course, the success of these treatments will depend on the reaction group to which the patient belongs. For the so-called positive reaction patients, the longer interval will not be a disturbing factor, but rather, even normal. Likewise, greater intervals must be maintained for normal or positively reacting patients with acute exacerbation of a chronic complaint. This is particularly true of relapses of sciatica. If the first treatment is followed by distinct improvement (reduction of symptoms by 75% or more), one should wait with the second treatment until the condition begins to worsen again. Should that fail to happen, no further treatment should be performed, even if the patient insists. At first glance this last statement seems somewhat odd. However, in a large practice, you will soon see that patients have the tendency to want to continue treatment when it is no longer required. Sometimes, complaints are even simulated or exaggerated just so that further treatment is given. This may be explained by acupuncture's regulative action on the vegetative nervous system. The patients find themselves in a better overall condition; they are more balanced mentally and feel physically good. In such cases, maintain a healthy firmness and do not let the reins slip out of your hands. After the desired effect has been achieved, too many treatments do more harm than good.

The Duration of Therapy

The Duration ofTherapy: Subjective and objective freedom of complaints should serve as your main guideline. If improvement is slow, you should increase the treatment intervals to two weeks as soon as the first significant improvement has been perceived. Should the longer interval prove to be beneficial, it may be increased to three and four weeks as soon as possible. A total of 15 treatments should not be exceeded, except in special cases such as paralysis, etc. If no desired results have been achieved by that time, you are either dealing with a non-responder or an irreversible disorder which is not accessible to acupuncture. If only a slight, positive result is achieved, you should still discontinue treatment for two to three months, after which time treatment can be resumed in the usual manner.

In summarizing, we can say that the normal interval between treatments is 5-7 days, and should only be reduced or increased in exceptional cases. There seems to be a correlation with normal wound healing. A total of 15 subsequent treatments should not be exceeded. The length of the intervals between treatments should be increased after an improvement has been seen. In this way, treatment is not discontinued abruptly, but gradually. Whenever possible, follow up of cured cases is not only desirable for statistics and documentation, but also for purely medical reasons.

Warning!

Has a patient received x-ray or radium therapy, acupuncture treatment should not be commenced until 6 months to one year thereafter. Irradiation has a blocking effect, rendering effective acupuncture treatment impossible. The same applies to spa therapy and the subsequent reactions thereto; one to two months must elapse prior to acupuncture treatment. The points G 3, K 6, SP 6, and B 31 must not be needled on the first days of a menstrual period, nor on women with complicated pregnancies.

Furthermore, the potency of some drugs is enhanced when taken while the patient is undergoing acupuncture treatments; digitalis, in particular, may have a faster cumulative effect than usual. Contrasexual hormones (e.g. androgens in women) may limit acupuncture's action to a great extent; cortisone less so. The same applies to thyroid depressants. In acupuncture analgesia, the effect is reduced or delayed if the patient has been conventionally premedicated.

Chapter VI

INDICATIONS FOR ACUPUNCTURE

Having discussed all the important theoretical aspects of acupuncture, we now turn to its practical application. We especially want to discuss the disorders which offer the beginner a good chance of achieving desired results and with which he should start. We recommend beginning with simpler disorders and not, as is unfortunately quite common, with an especially complicated case. It is understandable that a critical physician wants to be quickly convinced whether or not it is worth his while to learn acupuncture at all, and therefore attempts to test all that has been said herein on one of his more difficult cases – who may be resistant to therapy or even unresponsive. But he has not yet had the necessary experience, and hence, is apt to fail. However, he rarely seeks the source of error in himself, but rather simply rejects the method, thereby doing himself more harm than good.

Now, let us classify the individual disorders. Group I includes conditions which are relatively easy to influence; II includes those which are more difficult and less promising; III includes those which require considerably more effort. The beginner should limit himself to Group I at first, even though there too, as always in medicine, there may be negative exceptions. The locations of the points mentioned below and the range of symptoms for which they can be used will be described later on.

Although the above aspects should be given preference both for teaching purposes as well as in the sense of the ever-necessary individual therapy (which cannot be replaced by "cookbooks," that is, standard point combinations), I still wish to begin with the description of the disorders which are the most accessible to acupuncture in order to increase your interest in the method and give you all the more reason to learn the points and the corresponding symptoms, tiresome as that may be. Let us start at the head.

Cephalalgia: The information in the chapter on pulse diagnosis also applies here; that is, the point combinations listed below are only guidelines, and cannot be used under certain circumstances if the pulse reveals a distinctly different indication. Nevertheless, you will have an easier time in the beginning if you use such proven combinations and revert to others only if they fail. Furthermore, the metals listed here only represent general recommendations, and are not to be considered as absolute rules. This data is presented so that points which are usually acupunctured with gold needles are followed by "(gold)". If this is not specified, then silver, or perhaps steel needles are to be used. Cephalalgia

Acupuncture's primary aim in all types of cephalalgia is to normalize the vascular activity in the head. This can be achieved in various ways. Should there be a general weakness of the circulatory system – which always reveals itself in an altered (usually in the sense of YIN) pulse finding at the pulse point for Pericardium – we use the points P 6 or 7 (gold). If a hormonal disorder is present, especially in women – this usually revealing itself in the pulse of the Kidney, Liver, and Spleen-Pancreas – we use K 8 (gold) instead or as adjuvant. As we know from the description of the flow of energy, this point is located on the inner side of the lower extremity. A point for the head on the leg: You, the reader, will no longer be surprised by this. Expect your patients to be, though. Mild headaches of strictly vascular origin may be approached via the point 3H 4; indeed, even just massaging this point with the finger can bring about rapid (short-term) disappearance of pain. This is often a significant diagnostic clue. The points for regulation of the cerebral vessels are more local in position. Our nomenclature refers to longitudinal and transverse flow. For the former, the following points should be considered: PV 19, PV 16, PdM.

Once again, these points lie on one of the two "vessels" and do not have partners like the points on the meridians do. Therefore, each point requires only one needle, whereas points on meridians require two: one on the right and one on the left side of the body. For transverse flow, the point G 3 should be considered (thus, bilaterally). To directly influence the vegetative system, use the point B 10, thereby stimulating the vagus (parasympathetic nerve); for the sympathicus, G 20. This is the foundation for headache treatment. There are also numerous factors and secondary influences to be taken into consideration, for example, residual conditions from sinus inflammations in patients with frontal headache. Here, the points B 1 and 2, as well as G 14 are of major importance. For pain on the crown of the head, we must always consider the possibility of the intestinal function being disturbed. Therefore, in these cases, we will use the points LI 4 (gold) and/or SI 3. However, disorders of the intestinal tract remind us of the above-stated regarding the pulse. Basically, the treatment of headache is the same as that of migraines. Here, however, a strong vegetative component must be taken into consideration, which we can treat not only with the two main points, B 10 and G 20, these influencing the vegetative system, but also with the combination CV 15 and PV 19, thereby taking the possibility of psychologically influencing the vegetative system into account, and thus treating the cases simultaneously from both aspects. *Bachmann* once very appropriately called this combination the "Bellergal® (belladonna) of acupuncture", which describes its effect very well indeed. Distinct worsening due to weather changes, or actual dependence of the attacks on the latter, is treated with the point 3H 15, or better yet, it is used as adjuvant.

Migraines

Migraines: Some interesting data from *Abele* distinguish different migraine types, and thus present further aspects on which point selection may be based. His data are based on the description of the migraine attack's onset. He defines three groups:

1. True hemicrania. This classical migraine phenomenon usually shows a change in the pulse in the sense of YIN in the region of the Gallbladder and Bladder, while Kidney and Liver are usually in a YANG state. The points which that author mainly recommends are G 43 and 40 (gold), B 64 and 67 (gold), and B 2 and 3, G 4 and 17 as well as K 1.
2. A group characterized by pain beginning in the neck and radiating over the head to the eye. These complaints can appear unilaterally or bilaterally, but must be considered as a form of migraine because of their attack-like appearance. In these cases, the Large Intestine Meridian pulse is usually altered in the sense of YIN, and the Kidney Meridian pulse in the sense of YANG. The points indicated for this group are especially LI 4 and SI 7 (gold), as well as B 1, 2, and 4, and K 1 and 3, perhaps also 6.
3. Finally, another group is distinguished, in which the pain and attack usually start bilaterally in the temple region. Here, we see an alteration of the pulse in the sense of YIN in the Stomach and Small Intestine; YANG pulses are found in the Heart Meridian. The main points for this group are: SI 4, St 36, and 41 (gold), as well as H 3 and St 1 and 2.

All these groups have a point in common, which should be taken into consideration: B 60. This is acupuncture's main point for all types of pain, especially pain in the long back musculature. That is why this point is indicated particularly for the so-called cervical migraine, used together with PV 13.

Now, you will certainly say that hithertofore, I limited the maximum number of needles per treatment and now present a whole score of points, the sum of which far surpasses this number. However, the latter are only meant as an extensive catalogue. We never use all of these points at the same time. In the first session, we only use a basic combination of points indicated by the patient's case history and symptoms, if we have not arrived at different conclusions via the pulse. If, after the first or first few treatments, these combinations do not lead to, or only partially achieve, our aim, the other points listed, or those indicated by the pulse findings are to be used. The same applies of course to all the other conditions to be described. At this point, allow me to make another general comment. Occasionally, for example in headaches or migraines, complete cure or even noticeable improvement is not achieved. However, the attacks can almost always be shortened or the pain reduced. Simultaneously, a phenomenon appears which I have already briefly mentioned. Drugs which have become ineffective prior to the onset of acupuncture therapy suddenly regain their potency. In general, all simultaneously

administered medication, even that given for other disorders, has a stronger effect under acupuncture. This can be observed particularly in the effect of digitalis; much less so in insulin administration and similar substitution therapy. Only hormones (cortisone to a slight extent; sexual hormones to a much greater extent) and thyroid depressants are exceptions. In these cases, simultaneous acupuncture treatment should be discouraged as a rule; it must always be avoided following x-ray or radium therapy. In the one case I have observed after atomic radiation, no acupunctural effect could be established either. I cannot say to what extent these cases were non-responders as such. Therefore, prior to treating any new case, you must find out what drugs or medication the patient has been taking. Chronic consumption of painkillers is unfortunately very common among headache sufferers. Heavy smoking and alcohol abuse can also distinctly reduce acupuncture's efficacy. The dosages of other medication must be reduced in agreement with each patient's family physician or specialist after the first improvement has been achieved via acupuncture. Usually, the reduced consumption of medication is the first sign that an effect has taken place, expecially in headache cases.
Evaluation: Cases of cephalalgia and migraine usually belong in Group I (see beginning of this chapter); about 30% in Group II. If all of the above-mentioned influential factors have been properly taken into consideration, cephalalgia and migraines will rarely fall into Group III.

Disorders of the Ear, Nose and Throat

Disorders of the Ear, Nose and Throat: In discussing frontal headache, I have already mentioned its correlation with sinus inflammations. Symptoms of this type also frequently appear postoperatively. Usually, the point LI 19 is added to the above combination. This point, like the entire meridian itself, has a strong influence on mucous membrane, especially on the nasal mucous membrane. And we also know – from data of *Gross,* and *Majer,* for example – just to name two – that this point represents an important reflex zone. Acupuncture does not touch the mucous membrane directly, but has a very extensive action thereupon via many points. Furthermore, for all sinus inflammations, the point PdM, which lies on the Pilot Vessel, in the middle of the bridge of the nose, is used. This point, needled together with B 1 and/or 2 with silver, has an extensive action on sinus inflammations.

Hay Fever

Hay Fever: Here, too, the point LI 19 can be used successfully, together with the points B 1 and 2, G 3, PdM (silver), as well as LI 2 or 3 and/or 4 (gold). Treatment should already be completed before seasonal attacks are to be expected, and must therefore be performed during the attack-free periods. Acupuncture is also effective during attacks at times, however, only freedom from attacks during the usual periods is true proof of its effect.
Evaluation: Sinus inflammations usually belong in Groups I and II, whereby free breathing through the nose immediately after the first treatment is prognostically important. Postoperative inflammations have a lower rate of efficacy and often show recidivation.

On the other hand, only a small percent of hay fever cases belong in Group I; they are usually found in Group II; not infrequently in III as well.

Tinnitus

Tinnitus: Tinnitus represents the greatest crux of all ear, nose, and throat disorders. Tinnitus comprises a large percentage of cases both in private practice and in outpatient clinics. There are many types of treatment; the effect thereof is relatively slight. During my years at the ENT Department of the Policlinic Hospital of the City of Vienna (Head: Prof. *E.H. Majer,* M.D.), I treated a great many such cases and was also able to do follow up studies. Even acupuncture achieved a very limited success rate in comparison to its usual efficacy, nevertheless, this rate is still distinctly higher than that achieved with other methods. Here, I would like to add that those cases which are usually resistant to conventional therapy react especially well to acupuncture. The same goes for all disorders with the exception of malignant growths. Still, tinnitus clearly belongs in Group III and cannot be recommended to the beginner, not lastly because in these cases, other causes are often decisive and can only be discovered, if at all, if one has had a lot of experience with pulse diagnosis. Points are 3H 23, SI 18, G 3, 17, and 19. P 6 or 7 are usually added (gold).

Trigeminal Neuralgia and Facial Paralysis

Trigeminal Neuralgia and Facial Paralysis: Again, two different disorders are dealt with together. This is often the case in acupuncture. In this treatment, the tensest zones, that is, local and personal points, are very important. They are easy to find by gently stroking the skin. They are always acupunctured with silver needles, just 2 mm deep, and often immediately release an attack in trigeminal neuralgia patients, which is why you must make them aware of this unpleasant fact ahead of time. Usually, the attack disappears as rapidly as it appeared and is replaced by a comfortable warm feeling, the outward manifestation of which is an especially pronounced formation of red halos around the inserted needles. The following general points are administered in addition: SI 3 and 18, St 1, 4, and 7; 3H 23, G 3. 3H 5 is usually acupunctured with gold needles.
Evaluation: Trigeminal neuralgia usually falls into Groups I and II; facial paralysis rather into Groups II and III.

Vertigo

Vertigo: Cases of vertigo are quite common. Here, you should only take on patients who have been examined by an ENT specialist and have revealed no irreversible conditions. I would like to mention one form right away for which treatment is always successful and easy to perform: Dizziness from looking upwards. It can usually be eliminated immediately with only one treatment. The point CV 6 (gold) is used. This is a good point for beginners, who will quickly learn to trust acupuncture by using points like this one for certain disorders, and thus increase their motivation to continue studying. Naturally, CV 6 also plays a dominant role in the treatment of all other cases of vertigo, together with SI 5 and St 18, G 3 and 20; B 2 and 10; 3H 23.

The same points are to be considered for the treatment of *Menière's* disease.
Evaluation: Vertigo usually belongs in Groups I and II; *Menière's* disease rather in Group II to III. In these cases, great attention should also be paid to the pulse diagnosis.

Ophthalmology

Ophthalmology: We only use acupuncture for a few indications in this field. Blepharospasm is the most common. Here, too, we very often find local and personal points to be the most important treatment component. As in trigeminal neuralgia, they are found by palpating the tense areas. The general points are the same as for treatment of hay fever. Here, it is often necessary to apply the above-described fastened or "permanent" needles using adhesive strips to keep them in place for hours or days at a time. These special, thumbtack-like silver needles must be frequently checked as to position and reaction; use thereof must remain limited to patients who are responsible, observant, and stay in touch with the physician. As to other disorders of the eye, only nonspecific inflammations such as choroiditis, for example, can be considered for acupuncture treatment. Here, too, the results acupuncture achieves are not very spectacular, but are definitely comparable to repetitive cortisone therapy.
Evaluation: I would classify both above-mentioned disorders in Group II in milder, recent cases, and III in chronic cases.

Mental Illness

Mental Illness: True mental diseases should be excluded from acupuncture even if for no other than forensic reasons. Likewise, hysterics, hypochondriacs, and depressive patients should be referred to the appropriate specialist. Certainly, one may find individual cases in the last group, which can definitely be treated successfully with acupuncture. However, I only approach cases of this kind together with experienced psychiatrists or neurologists, or better said, upon their request. The beginner often tends to treat any case which has proven resistant to other forms of therapy mainly to prove acupuncture's effectiveness to himself. Often he is also forced by the public, which believes that spectacular results in other or similar illnesses can be achieved in all disorders. Depressive states within the frame of other disorders are frequently eliminated. However, in my opinion, this can be mainly traced to the fact that patients in pathological conditions, especially those of long standing, fall into a state of gloomy resignation and no longer expect any improvement. If, however, acupuncture achieves improvement, the patient becomes euphoric, this favorably influencing the rest of the healing process. Now, if the word depression or depressive appears anywhere in the case history of a patient of this type, he arrives at the conclusion that he had two independent illnesses at the same time and recommends acupuncture to friends suffering, for example, from endogenic depression. However, the chances of achieving any kind of effect on endogenic depression with acupuncture are extremely slight. Not only that, but you may then be faced with the forensic situation of a patient attempting or even succeeding in committing suicide. So, hands off psychiatric cases, especially schizophrenia, hebephrenia, endogenic depression, psychoses and other similar disorders.

We have to give another matter some thought. Earlier I said that acupuncture influences the vegetative nervous system's equilibrium. This goes hand in hand with a marked improvement in mental balance resulting in a general feeling of well-being. This explains the astounding tendency of many patients to want to continue acupuncture treatment when it is no longer required, especially when so-called "psychologically tonifying or sedation points", or better expressed, "psychologically harmonizing points" are often administered. These are: H 3, 5, 7; St 36, CV 6, 15; PV 4, 11, 13, 16, and 19, just to name the most important. St 36 is also called "Godly Equanimity", which is descriptive of the state its repeated use achieves; a state which we modern humans in this age of stress so sorely need. Therefore, the above-mentioned tendency is understandable, but it should not persuade the physician to continue therapy longer than necessary upon the patient's request. I again refer to what I stated before: Too many not absolutely indicated treatments can destroy an already manifest positive effect.

Sexual Disorders

Sexual Disorders: A lot of attention is given to sexual disorders, especially in classical works on acupuncture. Today as well, disorders of this type are not at all rare, even if they are not always expressed directly. You will stumble upon them much more frequently in probing case-taking, especially in disorders such as migraines, gastritis, colitis, etc. Here, we especially find ejaculatio praecox, impotentia coeundi, deficient or exaggerated libido, etc. suitable for treatment. Points to be considered are: St 30 and 36; K 6, CV 4 and 6, less frequently 1 and 2, as well as PV 4 less frequently 1 and 2. Depending on the type of symptoms, the majority of these points are acupunctured with gold needles (in cases of hypofunction) or with silver needles (hyperfunction). Of course, you will also have to employ points having a pronounced hormonal action. These are B 31 (especially for women) and PV 16 for both sexes.

These disorders in particular usually go hand in hand with psychological stress. Therefore, the above-described points must also be considered. Depending on the symptomatology, they are needled with gold or silver, or the points are selected according to their indications. Also, we must not forget the so-called "Bellergal® of acupuncture", (CV 15 and PV 19). Especially these sexual disorders often appear as the basis of the illness which appeared first after the latter has been cured. This has already been mentioned. If disorders of this type can be causally connected with the conditions expressed originally, they must always be treated in conjunction therewith.

Evaluation: Usually Group I, less frequently II.

Mental Instability

Mental Instability: When treating cases of mental – as well as vegetative – instability in the presence of actually mild somatic and functional disturbances, acupuncture points for the psychological disorders must be included in the program accordingly. This of course applies to treatment of the sexual disorders discussed above, as well as when the patient's personality shows it to be necessary. The physician finds this type of instability much more frequently in the form of stagefright or fear of examinations. For these cases, we prefer to use the points H 3 (gold) and H 5 and 7 as main points. Further, B 15, P 6, LI 4, as well as CV 6 and 15, and PV 19 are added as supplements.

In my opinion, the frequently-heard complaints of complete nervous exhaustion, lack of energy, of easily becoming mentally exhausted, and irritability also belong in this group. All of the above-mentioned points can be considered here; in addition, SP 2, 4, 5, 6 and 9, as well as Li 9. Another point, which is also capable of giving the patient initiative is B 39. It is especially important for weak concentration, together with P 6 and 9, as well as PV 19. Anxiety, especially at night, is an important factor in all of these conditions. A special point for this is P 9. For nightmares, which are often an expression of anxiety in children, the point is St 44. *Evaluation:* Mental instability almost always belongs in Group I; rarely in Group II. Therefore, it represents a good indication for the beginner, even if the positive results achieved can only be determined subjectively.

Insomnia

Insomnia: There is a classical combination which serves as the foundation for treatment of this disorder: K 6 (gold) and B 62 (silver), likewise PV 19. In the majority of cases, these points form the framework of insomnia treatment. The selection of more points depends on the pulse, as well as particularly on the so-called influential factors.

Thus, you may encounter insomnia resulting from a general weakness particularly in mentally lethargic individuals. St 36 is then added as well as SP 2. Disturbances of the functioning of the stomach, even in the absence of complaints, require CV 13. A similar disorder in the lower intestinal tract requires the point 3H 10. Chest congestion, or often only slight stasis or edematous alterations in the thoracic organs, can be favorably influenced via Lu 9. In this brief discussion of the treatment of insomnia, the principle of seeing and thus treating the individual as a whole appears again. The frequent complaint of cold feet, also during the night, fits in here too. Unfortunately, little attention is paid to complaints of this type in our Western medicine. Here, focus is on the points SP 5 and K 8. Of course, all these main points for specific influential factors are not only effective in the treatment of insomnia, but rather, are also indicated for all other corresponding influential factors in other disorders. Contra-indications are extremely rare; criteria thereof are not yet important for the beginner, who should proceed by discontinuing the use of what he believed to be correctly selected points in regard to the specific influential factors if they produce no reaction after several treatments. After renewed, more exact exploration of the patient, he may discover new aspects, or limit himself to the fundamental treatment of insomnia, thereby deleting treatment of the influential factors completely or temporarily.

The opposite of insomnia, somnolence, especially during the daytime, should also be mentioned. The points are G 23 and 24, St 18, and SP 5.

Spastic Disorders

Spastic Disorders: Let's turn briefly to spastic disorders. *Parkinson's* disease is practically inaccessible to acupuncture, therefore there is not much point in treating parkinsonians therewith. Likewise, I do not recommend acupuncture treatment of epilepsy, better said, grand mal. However, absentia epileptica (a form of petit mal epilepsy) frequently responds very well, especially in children or recent cases, and represents a good indication. The points are: B 2, 8, 10; G 20, CV 15, PV 11, 19, and 20. This transient loss of consciousness in conjunction with general disorders is often seen in children who do not suffer from petit mal: general developmental disorders, asthenia, weak concentration, children who tire easily, anorexia, etc. All of the following points should be considered for complex cases of this type: B 39, LI 4, PV 6a, 9, 10, 11, 11a, 13, 13a, and 19. If the disorders are mainly somatic and the psyche plays only a subordinate role, the so-called metabolic points (according to *Bachmann*) should be considered. This refers to adult patients as well.

Metabolic Points

Metabolic Points: These are B 54 and 58, K 2 and 6; Li 13, LI 2, 3, and 4. These points are extremely important in the overall treatment of the patient. They can often be used in the first sessions when, despite the case history and examinations, no definite cause for the complaints can be determined for the moment – also if the pulse finding is unclear – making it difficult to decide where to start. We can make no mistakes with these points because they call forth a balance or equilibrium of the individual metabolic factors, this always having a positive effect.

These metabolic points are extremely important and are part of the mandatory framework of every treatment, for example, of the skin, or digestive disorders.

Pain: Let us now turn to a new field, pain. First of all, a few general comments. There are pain perception centers on the skin which may coincide with acupuncture points, and sometimes even lie on a meridian, but whose locations are not identical to those of acupuncture points; they are often found outside the meridians. We call them personal points, ("points personelles") or spontaneous points. They must always be included in any treatment of pain if indicated exactly by the patient. This purely local needling of a spontaneously painful point or the punctum maximum of a spasm, usually with a silver needle, is called "locus-dolendi" needling. However, aside from these local, spontaneous pain points, there are several very important general points for the treatment of pain: The main point for all types of pain, regardless of location or duration, is B 60. It is always given as a supplement, especially if no progress is made with local or specific treatment. Li 2 and 3 should be selected for all types of spastic pain. 3H 5 and B 23 should be considered for all types of rheumatic pain. If pain is intensified by dampness, cold, snow, rain, or wind, the point 3H 15, which *de la Fuye* called the "hygrometric point" should be considered. If pain "migrates", that is, continually changes its location, or even alternates segments or sides, the points G 38, 40 and 43 are recommended. G 38 is also indicated for the quite common complaint of "pain all over", having no real punctum maximum. In these cases, the points K 6 and 3H 10 can also be added as supplements. Thus, the points mentioned above are used for the following situations:

1. If no precise picture is obtained despite an exact case history, examination, and pulse control. The first specific aspect is usually revealed after one or more treatments using the above points, and should then be approached specifically. Whether one, several, or all of the above points are then used in further sessions will depend on the progress of the treatment in each individual case.
2. One or more of the above points may be used as supplements in very specific treatments as well, be they based on the pulse or on the indications.
3. They must always be used (individually or together) if they are located where the pain is perceived strongest.

Toothache: Aside from all these general main points, there are also many specific main points, for example, LI 1 for toothache or in dental surgery. Any experienced acupuncturist sitting in a dentist's chair constantly massages this point on the lower inner corner of the nail of the index finger, just outside the cuticle, with another fingernail during the entire unpleasant procedure. It's worth the effort. Of course, this does not mean that one should neglect caring for ones teeth, but there are enough situations where this point is useful (I'm speaking from my own experience!).
Evaluation: Group I to II.

Intercostal Neuralgia: The main point for intercostal neuralgia is P 7. Aside from this point, which should always be used throughout the course of therapy (gold as a rule), there is also a very effective local constellation. Silver needles are inserted along the painful zone on the upper and lower edges of the affected ribs, 3-4 fingerbreadths apart from each other. Gold needles are inserted ventrally and dorsally on the juncture of the costal cartilage and rib bone.
Evaluation: Positive results, usually Group II.

Other main points of this type are: 3H 5 for any pain in joints (also non-rheumatic); SP 2, 3, and 5 for all types of "pain in the bones"; B 31, 54, 58, and 60 for lumbago, sciatica, etc.

Now, let us turn to the typical treatment of various, common painful conditions and describe a basic method, with which even the beginner cannot go wrong as a rule. At the most, he will fail if he does not deal with each basic, individual causative factor, these only revealing themselves in the course of treatment. I have often stressed this before. Therefore, please do not ever use my data like a "cookbook", but rather just as a foundation, which, indeed, will be sufficient in many cases.

Pain in the Upper Extremities

Pain in the Upper Extremities: Let us begin the discussion of pain with the upper extremities. The points LI 10, 11, and especially 15 are main points for all pain in the whole upper extremity no matter if caused by a simple muscle spasm, an inflammation, or spastic paresis. SI 4 and 9, 3H 5, Lu 5, and LI 4 are also frequently used. If the patient perceives pain predominately or only when he lifts his arm to the side, the points LI 13 and 14 are used as main points. If it is difficult for him to move his arm to the back (for example, the patient is unable to tie apron strings), these points are replaced by SI 9. If pain is limited to, or predominately in, the lower arm, SI 7, 3H 5, Lu 7, and especially LI 10 are mainly used. The main points for the hands and fingers are SI 5, 7, and Lu 11.

Joints of the Upper Extremities

Joints of the Upper Extremities: If mainly the joints of the upper extremities are afflicted, the point selection varies in part. The main points are: 3H 5, B 58, G 38, and SP 5, perhaps B 23 as well. Of course, here, we must not lose sight of the influential factors, which have already been discussed in detail. If the shoulder joint is the most affected, the main points are LI 4, 11, 14, 15, 16, as well as 3H 15. Naturally, the points mentioned in the foregoing sections concerning impaired movement in different directions are also valid here. For the elbows we recommend SI 4, Lu 5, and LI 11; for the hands, the same with the addition of Lu 9. We advise using 3H 3 and 5, as well as SI 4 for the joints of the fingers. For these small joints, a method which has already been discussed, the Ou-Rou method, is frequently used. This method consists of rapidly pricking or penetrating the skin with the needle once on each lateral and medial end of the skin fold of all interphalangeal joints. In this method, the needle is not left in the tissue, but rather, it is immediately removed again. This procedure is quite painful for the patient, but usually brings considerable relief and improved mobility, often already at the physician's office. Vessels over the joint at these end points of the skin furrow must be avoided. If performed properly, there should be no bleeding.

Paresis (Upper Extremity)

Paresis (Upper Extremity): In conjunction with the above, pareses and other disorders of the upper extremities shall now be discussed. Here, I want to stress again that in general, the needles are inserted significantly deeper for paresis (and paralysis) than in routine acupuncture. By gently turning it, insert the needle continually deeper until either a sensation similar to an electric shock or an intense feeling of warmth along the meridian, usually in a caudal direction, is perceived by the patient. I have already discussed this technique, and have said that these sensations are also extremely valuable for prognosis. The main point for the entire upper extremity is LI 15, for both spastic and atonic paresis, as well as for hemiplegia, as long as the condition is not of longer standing than two years. This point is combined with LI 10 and 11; SI 4, P 7, and K 7. The main points for paresis of the hand are SI 4 and 7; 3H 3 and 5; LI 5, 10, and 11; as well as Lu 7. Weakness and limited mobility of the joints of the hand from paralysis or fracture, especially after a cast has been removed, are noteworthy. The point 3H 4 is used in these cases. When a condition of this type is limited to, or concentrated in, the thumb and index finger only, we add LI 6. The so-called writer's cramp, which is actually quite common, is another special affliction of this region. As a rule, it can be favorably influenced with SI 4 and 3H 5, as well as with the points listed above for the joints of the fingers, however, the Ou-Rou method is never used. Finally, we have paresthesia and the common complaint of cold hands. Here, the most important points are Lu 9, Li 3, P 6, 7, and 9. There are also three points on the palm of each hand, which do not lie on meridians, which are used. They are not difficult to locate and lie on the vola manus between the distal heads of the 2nd and 3rd, 3rd and 4th, and 4th and 5th metacarpals respectively. Needling of these points is very painful and the needles are usually inserted very superficially, but are left lying in the tissue somewhat longer. Intense red halos around the inserted needles appear very soon, pale rapidly, and later reappear to a

lesser extent. The fingers distal to these loci first turn a bluish, livid color which then changes to a healthy pink. This type of acupuncture treatment brings about a short-term anastomosis. The results which this form of treatment achieves are considerable.
Evaluation: All of the above-discussed disorders of the upper extremity can mainly be classified as Group I to II.

Now that we have discussed pain and related conditions of the upper extremities, I would like to delve into those of the lower extremities. The same sequence shall be maintained.

Points for the Entire Lower Extremity

Points for the Entire Lower Extremity: Again, first the most important points for the entire lower extremity: B 31, 60; G 30, 34; St 36, K 8, and all spontaneously painful points for "locus dolendi needling" as well. Here is a short description of the most important points: B 31 lies in the first sacral foramen and is one of the main points of every sciatica treatment. At the same time, this point has a strong, hormonally regulative action, especially in women, a fact which must always be kept in mind and of which the patient must be made aware. Needling B 31 may disturb the menstrual cycle. Usually, menstruation is delayed; indeed, it can even fail to take place, or intensity and duration thereof may be significantly changed. Therefore, do not use this point if the patient is menstruating unless absolutely necessary (severe, acute attack). The point also seems to influence the female libido in both the positive and the negative sense. We are already familiar with B 60 as the main point for pain. In general, G 30's main action is on the hips and pelvis. Especially in regard to the lower extremities, particular attention must be paid to the fact that when treating all localized joint or functional areas, the proximal and distal neighboring joints should always be treated as well.

G 34 is the undisputed main point for all disorders of the muscular system. Indeed, it will rarely be left out of a treatment program for the lower extremities. Aside from its psychological and vascular influence, which is of course also important here, St 36 also acts specifically on the legs. Its name ("Three Villages") indicates that it is able to increase walking capacity. Soldiers in ancient China supposedly had this point needled so that they would be able to march through three villages without tiring.

Finally, K 8's epithet, "Master of the Blood", also gives us an idea of what it does, that is, promote the blood supply all the way up to the pelvis. Regarding this point as well: Caution if the patient is menstruating or pregnant.

If we look at the lower extremity with regard to local pain, we also find specific points for individual areas: G 30, which has already been mentioned, for the thigh; B 58 and G 37, 38 for the lower leg; B 60 and 62 and K 1 for the entire foot. We like to use SP 5, Li 2, and K 7 for the dorsum of the foot.

Sciatica

Sciatica: Sciatica is the most common disorder of the leg. We differentiate high sciatic (B 31, 33, 34, 35, and 50; G 30); middle sciatic (B 54 and G 32); and low sciatic involvement (B 60), depending on which part of the leg is most affected. The results with acupuncture treatment are flabbergasting, especially in acute cases. There is usually immediate positive improvement after the first treatment and exacerbation after the second and third treatments. Therefore, I suggest testing whether or not the patient can accept still incomplete freedom from pain after the first improvement, and postpone further treatment. If pain again increases about one week thereafter, treatment must be continued, and the patient must take the negative reaction in stride. If pain subsides gradually, the process should be left to itself and not disrupted with more treatments. I have quite a few patients who come back for treatment every few years because of relapses of this type who are completely restored each time after only one treatment. Although they cannot be considered as truly cured, their affliction is under control and they have been helped. And that is the therapist's aim.

Inflammations of the Joints

Inflammations of the Joints: Now, let's turn to inflammations of the joints of the lower extremities. In general, the main points are: 3H 5 (the main point of all inflammatory, especially nonspecific conditions), SP 5 (the main point for all illnesses or disorders of the connective tissue); further, B 58 and G 38. Of course, all influential factors which we have already discussed must be taken into consideration, for example, weather (3H 15) or the so-called metabolic points, especially for nonspecific conditions. They are obviously able to produce a change, their scope of use thereby being broadened.

G 30 and B 54 (again the neighboring joint) are of particular interest as main points for the hip joint. Basically, processes in the hip are much more difficult to deal with than those in the knee. Arthritis of the knee responds well, even in chronic and therapy-resistant cases, and in my opinion, represents the main field of indication for acupuncture treatment of joints. The points are: B 54, Li 9, and G 34; perhaps also G 30 and 32, as well as St 36.

Bachmann also listed local points which have proven to be very effective, but which are not located on the meridians and are therefore left out of most acupuncture books. They are located 1) in the middle of the patella, 2) lateral and 3) medial to the lower edge thereof, and 4) in the midline of the extremity over the middle of the patella, about 2 fingerbreadths above its cranial tip; thus, a total of 4 points. I highly recommend these points, as well as the point SP 9. Here, I want to again stress that as a rule, at least the main points must be needled bilaterally, whereby the healthy or better side is needled first even for mainly unilaterally perceived and palpated pain or symptoms. I always proceed by needling each point first on the healthy, then on the affected side, and never needle all points on one extremity or side before turning to the other. According to the studies *Stacher* and I have made, which I briefly mentioned before, this seems to be the more effective method. I also always needle the main points first. In doing so, I have a target procedure right from the onset, therefore probably achieving better results as well.

For the ankles, ankle-joints, and joints of the foot, mainly the points B 54, 58, and 60 are used; perhaps also B 62, St 41, and K 6. Only the big toe has Li 3 as main point. Of course, the above-described Ou-Rou method can also be effectively used for the joints of the toes in the same manner and technique as for the fingers.

Paresis of the Lower Extremities

Paresis of the Lower Extremities: All the rules given above for the upper extremities are also valid for all types of paresis including peroneal paralysis. Thus, here too, the needle is inserted deeper and the release of a sensation similar to an electric shock, or a hot wave along the extremity is watched for. These phenomena also provide us with prognostic information as to the indication for acupuncture treatment. The most important points are: B 54 and 58; G 34 and 37/38, as well as St 36. G 43, K 3 and 7, as well as B 62 are also of interest as secondary points. Here too, the previously mentioned guideline concerning the duration of the condition is valid. That is, a paralysis of more than two years' standing hardly offers a chance of achieving desired results. In all types of paralyses, the individual treatments may be given more frequently – even daily. However, as soon as distinct signs of a positive change can be observed, treatments should only be given once a week, as otherwise done, and the patient instructed to exercise daily instead. Here too, my method is unconventional, especially for spastic paralysis. Classical exercises ("one and two and one and two...") brought very poor results in these patients. Proceeding from the fact that a person is more relaxed while playing a game (which is basically instinctive behavior), I have all such patients play ball without any set program. For the upper extremities, I simply have the patient pick up the ball and lay it down again in the beginning; later on, pass the ball from one hand to the other, and then throw it. If that works well, I let the patient do more complicated exercises like throwing the ball against the wall and catching it again, etc., and do not limit his imagination in any way. For the lower extremities, I have patients who are able sit on a chair facing the wall. Then I set up two boundaries (boards etc.) on the sides from the patient up to the wall, so that when kicked against the wall, the ball returns directly to his legs. The closer the chair is pushed to the wall, the faster the patient's reaction must be, the proximity being increased depending on the patient's ability. They enjoy these games because in a sitting position, they do not have the strain of supporting their weight and therefore see improvement much faster, this in turn greatly encouraging them psychologically.

Only then do I let them try exercises in rising from the chair and walking; if possible, at first during underwater treatment.

Circulatory Disorders of the Lower Extremities

Circulatory Disorders of the Lower Extremities: After this slight excursion into the field of physical medicine, it being essential for such cases, let us turn to circulatory disorders of the lower extremities, which represent a very good field for acupuncture. First, the predominately arterial disorders (as completely homogenous disorders are extremely rare). The most important point is SP 6 (also called K 8 or Li 5, as it is the point of intersection of the three YIN meridians of the lower extremity). It is also called the "Master of the Blood". Further, the points B 54, 58, and 60; G 34 and 40; St 36, and Li 2/3. Here, we also take into consideration the frequent complaints of cold feet, "crawling ants" in the lower legs, and cramps in the calf, which cannot be explained by local factors or fatigue. Practically the same points are used for venous disorders.

Varicose Veins

Varicose Veins: A word about varicose veins. Basically, on account of there being a tissular change, acupuncture cannot make varicose veins disappear. However, with the point SP 5 the accompanying pain may be eliminated immediately and for a long period of time. Acute thrombophlebitis is a contra-indication for acupuncture. Chronic recidivation may be approached via points promoting blood circulation plus SP 5, in particular, thrombophlebitis migrans, for which local points for similar indications should also be employed. The point SP 5 is the main point for "connective tissue weakness". We often see the triad: varicose veins, hemorrhoids, and vaginal and uterus prolapse. SP 5 is almost always acupunctured with gold needles according to the classical rules. In the beginning, we follow the guideline that the silver needle is mainly used for hyperfunction, cramps, pain etc.; the gold needle for hypofunction, weakness, etc. Apparent exceptions, such as gold for SP 5 for varicose veins, refer to the weakness of the venous wall, this representing the most essential aspect here. Therefore, if, prior to making any selection, you contemplate whether you are actually dealing with hyper or hypo, your decisions will not only be less mechanical, but more reliable and produce better results. Our modern patients, living under stress, will always require more silver needles. When in doubt, I always advise using silver rather than gold needles. Exceptions to this guideline shall always be mentioned.
Evaluation: Especially sciatica, osteoarthritis of the knee, and circulatory disorders belong in Group I. The other mentioned indications usually fall into Group II, less frequently Group I, and very rarely Group III.

The Digestive Tract

The Digestive Tract: The digestive tract represents a very important field for the use of acupuncture. Let's begin with the stomach. Again, first the main points. CV 13 is the main point especially for all types of cramps. The so-called Master Point of the Stomach is B 21. We will find these two points in almost all specific indications as well. For all types of stomach cramps, Li 13, B 60, as well as SP 2 and 3 are used in addition to the two above-mentioned points. For positive psychological influence, which is very important for such conditions, the point H 3 (gold) is added.

Gastritis

Gastritis: We like to use CV 12, 14, and 15; St 21 and 23, and often B 17 in addition to the already-mentioned main points when treating gastritis. The latter is the main point for action on the diaphragm, therefore, it is used for all conditions in which there is flatulence. If the above points do not achieve the desired effect for hyperacidity after several treatments, the point St 45 is occasionally added. This point is quite painful, as its name, "the gruesome payment", implies. For hypersecretory gastritis, it may be substituted with SP 3. Occasionally, I have seen improvement of hyperacidity with the use of St 41 and 42, but still have nothing against using appropriate substitution preparations, thus contributing to a more rapid improvement of such conditions.

Gastric and Duodenal Ulcers

Gastric and Duodenal Ulcers: I use practically the same points for ulcers as for gastritis. The chances of successful treatment are considerable. Of course, you will be able to convince yourself of the treatment's progress with x-rays and gastroscopy. Beginners are advised against treating bleeding ulcers with acupuncture. Indeed, encouraged by good results, one tends to treat all ulcer cases with the needle. And in view of the reports and all the literature thereon, one feels one can do so in good conscience. However, the goal and purpose of this book is to give the beginner a solid foundation with which he will never find himself faced with problems, especially not of a forensic nature.

In seeming contrast to what has just been said, allow me to call your attention to some data taken from an article by *Wehlend*. I have two reasons for this. First of all, *Wehlend* is a specialist in this field, and therefore, his statements are pertinent. For the treatment of ulcers, he uses practically the above-described points, whereby he generally limits himself to gold needles for the points CV 13, 14, and 15; and silver needles for St 23, at least in the majority of cases. Secondly, he treats fresh ulcers more frequently – about three times a week – until complete freedom from complaints is achieved and can be verfied by x-rays. Furthermore, he likes to have his patients lie under an electric heater during the treatment. Aside from the favorable effect of warmth as such for all abdominal processes, it relaxes the patient as much as possible, which is very important. He has come to the conclusion that a warm needle brings about better results. This opinion is completely justified, and was also presented in a preliminary communication by *Konnen* as well; it has, however, not yet been verified.

Needling causes a change in the stomach's tonus as well as in the dilation of the duodenum. In the latter case, x-ray detection of the presence of diverticula is thereby rendered possible. The above phenomena can be clearly verified by x-rays. Treatment should be discontinued when complete healing of the ulcer can be confirmed objectively. Subjective improvement is perceived much sooner, therefore, it is important to convince the patient to continue treatment even if he feels good. With this treatment, a special diet or reduction of alcohol or cigarette consumption is only required in exeptional cases.

Hyperemesis gravidarum

Hyperemesis gravidarum: This is another indication which can be quickly and successfully treated with acupuncture without harmful side-effects – which is particularly important here. Motion sickness or nausea can also be favorably influenced – ideally one to two weeks before travel by ship or plane is commenced. The required points are: Li 13 and 14, K 21, B 21, and St 21.

Treatment is similarly effective for heartburn. CV 21 ist the main point. When needed, the patient can also massage this point vigorously with his fingernail to bring about alleviation or disappearance of the complaints. The point St 12 can also be used as adjuvant.

Annoying hiccoughs can also be controlled successfully, even immediately after an operation. The points B 17 and 39, as well as St 12 and 21 are used.

Anorexia

Anorexia: This is another important indication, especially for children with extensive or complete lack of appetite. The three main points are: St 36 and 42, as well as Li 3. All three should be acupunctured with gold needles. If the small amount of spontaneously eaten food is also poorly digested or remains in the stomach for a long time, B 21 is added. After they have overcome their initial fear of the needles, children react well to acupuncture. However, especially in the treatment of children, the greatest attention should be paid to the influential factors mentioned. You must especially heed psychological factors as well as disturbed metabolism. Therefore, the metabolic points will have to be repeatedly used on children; more so than on adults.

Evaluation: The majority of the listed illnesses and disorders of the stomach and duodenum show good, often spectacular, results and therefore belong in Group I. Only rarely will a case fall into Group II. The above indications are especially suitable for the beginning acupuncturist.

Intestinal Disorders: In accordance with the precepts of the pulse, the Chinese distinguish between disorders of the large intestine and disorders of the small intestine, both of which may be spastic (YANG) or atonic (YIN). In daily practice, however, we almost always see disorders of both parts, because disorders very often influence other organs, especially in the digestive tract. Intestinal Disorders

Again, I want to list the main points at the beginning. They are: SI 3 and perhaps 8 as well; Li 2 and/or 3; LI 4, as well as CV 4. K 8 (gold) is recommended for regulation of the afflux of the blood.

Enteritis and Diarrhea: The main point for all types of diarrhea is SP 4. We like to combine it with Li 9 (gold). The latter point has a broad, general scope of action. Whenever this point is used, special attention must be paid to the influential factors. Some of the points listed for spasm can be added to this combination. Which one of them is selected depends on each individual case. Practice rapidly gives you a good idea of which points are best combined. Discussions with colleagues, such as those at congresses and meetings of individual acupuncture societies, are also very helpful. A general guideline for selecting the correct combination in these cases – aside from the pulse diagnosis – is that spasms which are not confined to the abdomen require the two Liver points. Li 2 should be given preference for somatic spasms; Li 3 for predominately mental tension. If the spasms are confined more to the upper abdomen, the points of the Small Intestine Meridian should be preferred; if they are in the colon, LI 4. If they are equally distributed in the small and large intestines, the point of choice is CV 4. Enteritis and Diarrhea

In treating enteritis and diarrhea, we must keep the influence of dampness and cold in mind. However, psychological states also play an important role. Many vernacular sayings acknowledge the connection. This goes not only for intestinal indications, but for most others as well.

Constipation: This is a complex field. Acupuncture treatment is very effective, especially for spastic constipation. It is clearly less effective for atonic constipation, especially habitual atonic constipation in women. The main points are the same for both: LI 4 and 10, less frequently 11, as well as SI 3. B 25, K 15, and St 25 are administered secondarily. For spastic constipation, these points are mainly needled with a silver needle and usually combined with Li 2 and 3 (as main spasm points). For atonic constipation, a gold needle is inserted into the above-mentioned main points. Furthermore, Li 9, G 34, and St 36 (gold) are added. The points CV 4 and 6 are also used quite frequently; the former usually with a silver needle for spastic constipation and the latter usually with a gold needle for atonic constipation. Again, the influential factors are extremely important. If the patient has severe meteorism at the same time (or it is the symptom of which he complains most), St 25, G 23 and 24, St 41, and SP 3 are indicated. Constipation

While undergoing acupuncture treatment, the patient should not take laxatives, especially not strong purgatives. He should use enemas instead. This is because bowels which are overly irritated from laxatives often react atypically, indeed even paradoxically when simultaneously stimulated by acupuncture. This is an important aspect, because it may be the reason for a point combination seeming to be ineffectual. Therefore, before you change the point combination, make sure that no laxatives are being taken at the same time, or have been taken immediately prior to acupuncture treatment. You need only change the originally chosen combination if the patient's denial of laxative consumption is reliable, should change not seem indicated for any other reasons.

Lastly, we take the same standpoint regarding hemorrhoids as regarding varicose veins. As they are the manifestation of complete structural change, we can expect no results from acupuncture.

On the other hand, in cases of the very unpleasant anal pruritus as well as anal eczema, the use of the points PV 1 and CV 1 (which are usually acupunctured with a heated needle), and SP 5, as well as the metabolic points, especially for anal eczema.

In concluding the discussion of the intestinal tract, we still must discuss the most important indication for acupuncture in this area.

Colitis

Colitis: Acupuncture is without doubt superior to conventional medicine in the treatment of this disorder. This applies to all types thereof. Spastic or mucous colitis are the most common. However, the more dangerous type, chronic ulcerative colitis, is not uncommon either. In acupuncture, both types are treated in the same manner. The most important points are: SI 3, Li 13, LI 4, St 21 and 25; CV 13 and 15. The stool usually normalizes after only four treatments following an exacerbation reaction, especially after the second and third treatments. The same is often true of the other types, and therefore, the patient must be informed accordingly prior to treatment.

Because colitis (like other illnesses such as asthma, migraines, etc.) shows a tendency to relapse, especially during the greatest seasonal changes (spring and autumn), it is a good idea to call the patient in for a check-up the following spring or autumn, even after treatment has been successfully completed. In this way, relapses can usually be avoided. External influences of great magnitude, which affect the patient psychologically or physically, may also cause a relapse. If the patients have been informed, they always come for a check-up in time. In such cases, we are performing true prophylaxis.

You will rarely have occasion to treat the dangerous acute ulcerative colitis. Acupuncture treatment can be effective there too, however, it should never be performed at home or in a private office, but always in a hospital. In such cases, the profuse bleeding or the consequences thereof are dealt with first with the points B 39, SP 4 and 5, as well as P 6 (gold). After the bleeding has ceased, and transfusions and other necessary measures have been taken, the above colitis therapy points are used.

Evaluation: Most intestinal disorders fall into Groups II and I. Only colitis is a definite Group I indication, and therefore, can be highly recommended to the beginner (with the exception of the acute, ulcerative form). Of course, influential factors, such as the effect of cold (SP 4), or mental trauma (PV 19), or a correlation with menstruation (K 8), or others which we have already discussed must be kept in mind.

Disorders of the Liver and Pancreas

Disorders of the Liver and Pancreas: In the treatment of disorders of the liver and pancreas, you must first observe the basic rules that acupuncture cannot perform miracles if structural change or destruction, such as in cirrhosis or diabetes mellitus, has taken place. However, there are many borderline cases in which, for example, there are only slight changes in the liver function tests, the liver is somewhat enlarged, there is a feeling of fullness, or the patient suffers from generally poor digestion due to insufficient secretion, etc. In all of these cases, we can usually obtain good results, particularly via the points Li 6, 9, and 13, as well as B 18 (all with gold needles). In treating these cases, you must never lose sight of the fact that not only the liver is involved, but, almost always the pancreas, gallbladder, and stomach as well. Therefore, the corresponding stomach points, such as B 21 and St 36, are always combined. Also, pancreatic function is almost always insufficient as well when the patient complains of great fatigue, especially during the daytime. Here, I suggest the points SP 2, 3, 5, and K 8, and also B 20.

Cholecystitis

Cholecystitis: Chronic inflammations of the gallbladder in particular are treated via the points G 25, 26, and 27; less frequently 28, as well as B 19. Just as in the treatment of biliary colic, mainly the points G 37, 38, 40, but also 14, as well as Li 3 are very valuable. In cholelithiasis, we must consider the fact that acupuncture causes a significant increase in the motility of the gallbladder. This can bring about elimination of the stones. If they are the right form and size, they are eliminated naturally. However, if they are jagged or are too large to pass through the ductus choledochus without causing complications, obstruction of the latter can result, making surgery necessary. Here, too, the patient should be made aware of the possibility of complications of this type arising.

Evaluation: Most indications in this field are found in Group II; to a somewhat lesser degree in Group I. Still, quelling a biliary colic just by using the needle alone is quite an experience.

If we observe the entire range of disorders of the upper digestive tract and glands, we find ourselves faced with such a vast number of points that it is easy to become confused. From experience, I recommend always adhering to the main points first, that is, those which are given at the beginning of each list of indicated points. Associated or concurring ("assentiment") points are listed for almost all indications as well, all of these being located on the Meridian of the Bladder, hence, on the back. Therefore, it is advisable to treat the ventral points in the first sessions, and then perform one treatment using the dorsal points only (that is, B 18-22), combined only with Li 9 (gold). This treatment can be repeated later. This suggestion is based only on practical considerations as to the most comfortable position for the patient. Of course, if the patient can be comfortably positioned accordingly, ventral and dorsal points may be treated at the same time.

Cardiac Disorders

Cardiac Disorders: Because we are unable to act directly on the heart muscle, the valve, and the conduction system, the list of our indications for the heart is short. We are mainly able to influence nervous complaints of the heart, such as palpitations, tachycardia, etc. The main points are H 5 and 7, with which we have become familiar in the treatment of stagefright. The points Lu 7 and 9 (gold) may be used for all types of congestion, as long as they are not the result of cardiac decompensation. We are also often able to achieve extensive and rapid positive results for the forms of stenocardia which correspond to angina pectoris spuria (and are much more common than angina vera), by using the above-mentioned points together with CV 14 and 15, as well as B 17 and 21. These points can also be of importance for diagnostic purposes. Positive results can be maintained with H 3 and 9 (gold). The same procedure is used for *Roemheld's* syndrome.

Vascular Disorders

Vascular Disorders: Blood vessels respond well to acupuncture. In the discussion of the lower and upper extremities, I have already mentioned the circulatory disorders of the hands and feet, and especially, some special methods as well. Here, let us discuss intermittent claudication, which has not yet been mentioned as such. Its main points are: B 58, 60, and 62; G 34, as well as SP 5 (gold), and especially K 8. We are able to observe a rapid increase in walking capacity, and the patient does not tire as quickly. The same applies to cases of obstruction of large vessels, even the iliac artery, albeit to a somewhat lesser extent. A recanalization seems to take place. Therefore, you can also try using the same points for dry gangrene. This is usually very effective and thus, amputation may be avoided. The expression of the harmonizing action on the vegetative system will of course be conveyed to the musculature of the vascular system, thus explaining these effect, because the vascular musculature is regulated by the vegetative nervous system. Proof of this hypothesis is the complete absence of any effect of acupuncture whatsoever if there is severe arteriosclerosis. In cases of this type, pulse diagnosis is impossible. Of course, acupuncture is powerless against arteriosclerosis itself.

Hypertension and Hypotension

Hypertension and Hypotension: According to what has been said above, we expect acupuncture to have a favorable effect on hyper- and hypotension. Hypertension offers the higher rate of success. The main points are: H 7, P 7, K 2, and St 36, all with silver needles. We usually achieve a lasting normotensive level quickly, as long as the patient has not already

adjusted physiologically to the higher blood pressure level. Of course, we can expect no significant action on renal hypertension. Treatment of hypotension is more difficult and tedious, The following points are used in particular: H 9, P 9, Lu 9, K 7, K 8, as well as St 36; all with gold needles. You must expect frequent treatments to be necessary.
Evaluation: More cardiac disorders will fall into Group II than Group I. The opposite is true of vascular disorders. Intermittent claudication in particular also provides the beginner with good results.

Hematology

Hematology: The title of this section is somewhat pompous for the few indications we can list in this field. However, especially this field still seems to offer acupuncture many possiblities for development. *Fleischhacker* and *Stacher* showed very marked effects on disorders in this group after fields of disturbance had been eliminated. *Schroeder* and *Bischko* were able to describe impressive results after acupuncture treatment of agranulocytosis caused by drug abuse. Uncomplicated anemia can also be treated with the same points. In these cases there is a rapid increase in erythrocytes (up to one million), especially after needling of the point B 39. B 39 is our main point for erythropoiesis and arterial blood. B 17 is responsible for coagulation disorders and venous blood. The patient should be lying down when either of these points are needled, especially the first time, since syncope is not uncommon. However, it can be rapidly reversed with H 9 and/or P 9.
Evaluation: Group II. Collaboration with a specialist is most desirable especially in this field. The beginner will mainly use B 39 in order to be convinced of acupuncture's effectiveness in the treatment of anemia.

Respiratory Tract

Respiratory Tract: Disorders of the respiratory tract represent a large field of indication for acupuncture. Several illnesses, such as sinusitis and hay fever, have already been discussed above in the section on ENT disorders. The according supplements and expansions shall be dealt with here.

Colds

Colds: The main point for the common cold is LI 4. It is usually acupunctured with a gold needle. However, treatment is only effective when performed during the period of time when the cold is first coming on. This is the period of time when the nose tickles and one is absolutely certain that a cold is imminent. By simply needling the point LI 4 during this timespan, which usually lasts about 20 minutes, development of the cold can be inhibited in the majority of cases. If this initial period is already over, acupuncture is less effective, indeed, often, no results can be achieved at all. Nevertheless, breathing through the nose can be facilitated, even if only for a short time. To that end, we use the points B 2, LI 20, and PdM. As already mentioned, the latter point (Point de Merveille) lies on the ventral midline over the bridge of the nose. It is called PV 25 in some books, although that is not exact. Aside from free breathing, strong secretion which may be tinged with blood follows, and then rapid improvement. The points for sinusitis are used instead of the above for chronic colds, however, points of both groups can be combined.

In general, we can use the main point, CV 17, for all disorders of the respiratory tract, including colds. It facilitates breathing and normalizes all pathological functions.

Pharyngitis

Pharyngitis: Lu 11, usually acupunctured with a silver needle, particularly influences complaints of the larynx and pharynx. Other points are B 1 and 12, G 2 and 3. The main point for combatting hoarseness, also caused by strain in speakers, singers, etc., is St 10. Aside from the latter, the other points are also used for various nasal disorders, such as ozena and anosmia. Here again we find a functional unit, which should be treated as such, that is, it should not be merely treated locally.

A less common indication for the pharynx is the sensation of an object being lodged therein. Endoscopy shows no such object, and the disorder can certainly be considered mainly psychological. However, it often leads to a change in the sense of taste, which can threaten the livelihood of people in certain professions. In these cases, psychological points, such as H 3 and St 36; CV 15 and PV 19 are added to the points mentioned above for the treatment of the nose and pharynx.

Bronchial Asthma

Bronchial Asthma: Acupuncture's main field of efficacy in the respiratory tract is bronchial asthma. Results achieved with acupuncture in bronchial asthma are so impressive, especially in children, that one wonders why it hasn't already become the treatment of choice. In selecting points, we always have to take the following into consideration: Bronchial asthma is a triad consisting of:

1. spasms of the bronchial tree with all of its branches. Therefore, spasmolysis is important;
2. an allergic factor, and
3. a psychological factor, that is, fear of an attack.

Furthermore, climatic, professional, and hereditary influences must also be taken into consideration although they can hardly be influenced.

Whichever of the three main factors predominates must be treated first. Here, I only want to list the individual specific actions achieved via the various points, which can all be combined with each other. They should be varied according to each individual patient and his progress.

The main point for any process in the thoracic region is CV 17, which I have already mentioned. The main point for the pulmonary region is B 13. In cases of spasm, they are acupunctured with silver needles. The local points for asthma therapy are Lu 1 and 2, St 13, and K 27. In order to combat the congestion present in each attack, Lu 7 or 9 is acupunctured, however with gold needles. The main point for the diaphragm, B 17, is administered for spasmodic breathing, impaired expiration or inspiration; usually silver needles are used. This achieves rapid and long-lasting facilitation of breathing. If the attacks come only, or especially, during certain weather conditions (fog, storms, etc.), 3H 15 is additionally acupunctured (gold). If there is putrid sputum or raised temperature, the main point for all inflammation, 3H 5, perhaps combined with B 11, is used.

The above points are especially effective for juvenile asthma, for which just about a 100% cure can be achieved. The points are the same for adults, however, the success rate depends on the extent and functional influence of simultaneously present emphysema. This guideline is also valid for prognosis: The more advanced the emphysema, the less results will be achieved. Severe thoracic deformities also play a negative role, as do extreme scoliosis, funnel chest, etc.

The influence of the psyche is significant in asthma in all age groups. To combat the fear of an attack, we use the points which have proven to be effective for psychological balance, H 3 and St 36 (gold); H 5 and 7; CV 15 and PV 19 (silver). As already said, the points can be combined with the spasm points of asthma therapy.

Before we turn to the third, allergic, factor, I would like to make one comment. We have already seen a close connection between the Large Intestine and Lung Meridians in the precepts of the pulse diagnosis. There, we established that these meridians are both responsible for elimination.

The Sequence of Elimination

The Sequence of Elimination: The following ancient Chinese saying illustrates what is meant. It refers to the ways of elimination and the sequence thereof in the body.

Whatever the kidneys and bladder cannot eliminate must be eliminated by the intestines. Whatever the intestines can no longer eliminate must be eliminated by the lungs. If all of them together cannot eliminate enough (toxins), then the skin must take over. And that which the skin can no longer eliminate leads to death.

One can contemplate this saying for a long time. It leads us directly into the ambiguity of the dynamic development of illness. It implies the body's attempt to regulate, which reveals itself in different ways; of a negative nature as well. Accordingly, not every fever is bad and must be suppressed. Vomiting and diarrhea can without doubt have a positive effect. A skin rash does not always have to be suppressed. Our predecessors know more about such things and made better use of that knowledge than we do today.

These processes are especially obvious in asthma. Thus, we see a strong correlation between constipation and diarrhea and asthma attacks. I once had a young farmer as patient, who suffered from asthma. He had had severe attacks since childhood and was also continually constipated. The asthma attacks could barely be influenced with drugs. Already after the first acupuncture treatment, this man had severe diarrhea, which the family doctor had a hard time treating. However, the asthma attacks, which would otherwise have been expected were absent. When he came to me again after about a week, I stopped the diarrhea with the point SP 4, with which we are already familiar. It worked like a flash, however, the next day, the patient had an asthma attack. After the following treatment, this time with asthma points, he got diarrhea again. The treatment continued with the reaction alternating between asthma and diarrhea, both of which became less intense from session to session until finally, after several treatments, both had disappeared, and have not recurred to date, that is, for several years. Therefore, not only in extreme cases like the one described must we take the processes in the intestines and the mucous membranes thereof into consideration both in the treatment of asthma and in the treatment of allergies as well.

We treat practically all allergic components of asthma via the points SI 3, LI 2, 3, and 4, as well as Li 13, that is, with several metabolic points. Also, the nose, a significant reflex zone as well as end point of the Large Intestine Meridian, must often be included in an asthma treatment program. The points are LI 19 and 20, PdM and B 2 or 1, with which we are already familiar. I do not want to neglect mentioning B 39, which also acts extensively on any process in the thoracic region, aside from its action on erythropoiesis. Finally, CV 21 and 22, which we also use for heartburn, are sometimes considered as supplements, and may also be combined with Lu 5 for a severe cough.

Again, we see the close connection between the respiratory and digestive tracts. This connection was already known of in the past, as can be inferred especially from the clear information from *Aschner*. In his "Lehrbuch der Konstitutionstherapie" (Textbook of Constitutional Therapy) he discusses the use of emetics, however, in enormous doses in comparison to the quantities common in our conventional cough remedies.

Here too, as in all my other suggestions for therapy, you must also consider any influential factors outside of this triad as well. In practice, you should first try a standard general treatment as given above. Of course, if other criteria are present from the start, a different initial procedure is indicated. If no results are achieved with the program selected, a type of therapy which varies from the normal or standard form and proves suitable can be developed on the basis of all other information, such as the pulse, influential factors, etc. An example as complex as asthma deserves the more detailed discussion of various ways with which it can be dealt. It stands to reason that an individual treatment is required in every case, however, it must be based on certain methods. If we have several different methods at our disposal, then a truly individual treatment is rendered possible. In other words, we don't just have one horse, but a whole team at our disposal. We can choose the leader, and replace him with another at will.

Evaluation: Acupuncture is effective for disorders of the respiratory tract. Asthma, particularly juvenile asthma, shows excellent results. Mainly in Group I, and especially suitable for a beginning acupuncture practitioner, not lastly because of the many combinations possible.

Skin Diseases

Skin Diseases: I find it important to turn to skin disorders at this point. Indeed, until recently, this has always been therapy's stepchild, and the most transgressions are still made in this field. This goes not only for the ladies, who contribute to the evil with indiscriminate use of various beauty aids, but also for the medical world, which is not always willing to see the skin as an important, if not **the most** important organ, but considers it only as an integument, a necessary covering for the body and its organs. However, if we recall the theory about the sequence of elimination, its great importance becomes clear.

Therefore, in treating all skin diseases, with the exception of venereal diseases, cancer, tuberculosis, and psoriasis (which very probably represents a negative hereditary factor, and being a constitutional factor, is therefore inaccessible to acupuncture), we mainly use the so-called metabolic points. Again, they are: B 54 and 58; K 2 and 6; Li 13, LI 2, 3, and 4.

In all cases of chronic dermatoses, the needle is inserted somewhat deeper than usual into B 54, whereby the exudation of a few drops of blood is desirable. We add 3H 5 for all recent, inflammatory skin diseases. All these points are almost always acupunctured with gold needles, as we must consider skin disorders as a weakness in the process of elimination and therefore tonify even if the condition appears to represent hyperfunction. Oozing or itching dermatoses are treated with B 47. For eczema, we like to combine LI 11 with some of the metabolic points.

Particularly when treating skin diseases, which are indeed an expression of maximum weakness, we always try to use a minimum of needles. Therefore, especially at the beginning of treatment, we combine only one metabolic point of a meridian at a time with the other appropriate points; for example, LI 4 with B 54 and K 2, but not LI 2 and 3 with B 54 and 58.

For severe pruritus with or without efflorescence, we use Li 6, LI 11, and B 13 (gold). The basic therapy for furunculosis is B 62, LI 11 and K 2 (silver); B 11 and CV 9 (gold). This can instigate the required change. For acne, LI 11 and K 2 are replaced by LI 1 and Lu 5.

Herpes Zoster: Herpes zoster requires special treatment. We use P 7 as main point (the main point for intercostal neuralgia), as well as B 60; we add H 3 (gold). Furthermore, we insert one silver needle into the middle of the most affected area, however, never into the efflorescence itself. Limit yourself to a maximum of 4-5 local needles. Extensive expediation of healing is usually achieved. In inveterate cases, the effect depends on the depth of the scars. If they go beyond a certain borderline, which however, varies from individual to individual, a positive effect cannot be expected. Herpes Zoster

Ulcers of the Leg: These too, require a special technique. K 8 is considered the main point. As it often lies within the ulcer, it cannot be used in such cases and must be replaced by SP 5 (gold for both). Li 9 is a supplementary point (also gold). Around the ulcer itself we insert about 6-8 needles spaced evenly in a circle in the transition zone between the callous edge and the striated border which has been altered by small, thrombosed veins. If there is slight bleeding, the area, including the ulcer, is covered with a nonirritant ointment, however, only if the ulcer is not covered with a soft, moist film. In the latter case, you can carefully cleanse the ulcer before treatment using a NaCl solution of slightly higher concentration. This therapy brings about very impressive and rapid healing. Ulcers of the Leg

Finally, we must also consider skin disorders in regard to their location, as well as the extent to which they are spread over individual areas of the body. We find that in general, the points LI 4 and 11, as well as Lu 5 are important for the head; PdM for the nose; St 45 for the lips. The neck requires SI 8; the axillae G 38 and 40; less frequently 43. The upper extremities are additionally influenced by LI 11; the lower by G 30, if these points have not already been included in the therapy. This data refers to all skin diseases on the specific areas mentioned. *Evaluation:* Because of the fact that the treatment of skin disorders implies a process of conversion, it is always of longer duration, and frequently, several adaptations of the treatment program are necessary. Hence, Group II, with the exception of ulcers of the leg, which belong in Group I (even used only unilaterally).

Urogenital Tract: Lastly, let us turn to disorders of the urogenital tract. We have already briefly discussed sexual disorders. The following conditions represent good indications for acupuncture. Urogenital Tract

Menstrual Disorders: First of all, the most important points for amenorrhea: B 31, St 30, K 8, CV 2, 3, and 4; PV 4 and 16, perhaps 2 as well. Gold needles are usually used. The important Mestrual Disorders points for dysmenorrhea are: B 31, K 13, 14, and 15; G 26, 27, and 28; CV 3. The main points for menorrhagia and metrorrhagia are: G 3, SP 6, and CV 6. The latter point also increases fertility in men, a fact of which you should make the patient aware.

All of the above-mentioned points are also suitable for treatment of leukorrhea. Because many of these points, especially K 8 and B 31, are also used for other indications (i.e. sciatica), the patient should be asked if there have been any such changes during acupuncture treatment of other ailments. In this way you can judge which points are especially suitable for indications of this type.

Likewise, all the above points have a strong action on impotence and frigidity, especially when combined with psychologically activating points and B 39.

As a side-note, I would like to list several points for colleagues who practice in the country which are able to accelerate the course of normal labor. These are B 60 and 67; K 6, as well as SP 5, and K 8. Maybe they can help some of you by shortening your night calls.

Kidney Disorders

Kidney Disorders: This is the field where acupuncture is least effective. In general, B 23 and K 7 may be considered for treatment. For nephritic colic, G 25, 26, and 27 can be effective. Stubborn cases of cystitis often react positively to B 27 and 28; K 2 and 6; as well as CV 4 and 6.

Enuresis nocturna in children – less frequently incontinence in adults – may respond well to Li 3, CV 3 and 4; SP 9, St 36, and K 2. The psychologically harmonizing points should be used for children. K 8 and CV 6 may also be used as supplements. Belongs to Group I.

Evaluation: All menstrual disorders fall into Group I. Treatment of kidney disorders won't bring anyone laurels; they fall into Group III.

We have now concluded the survey of the indications for and combinations in acupuncture suitable for the beginner. I again repeat that these suggestions are not a "cookbook", but rather, are meant to help the novice to become familiar with the material.

I am also including a list of the points discussed with their exact locations. Locating the points has already been discussed at the beginning of this book, and is not as difficult as it might seem at first glance once you have become familiar with the locations thereof. Of course, the list also includes the most important indications and is thus a type of recapitulation.

An anatomy atlas will certainly be helpful in studying the points and their locations.

Chapter VII

THE MOST IMPORTANT ACUPUNCTURE POINTS: LOCATIONS AND SYMPTOMATOLOGY

The sequence of the points now to be discussed corresponds to the traditional classification. The individual points are numbered in sequence along the corresponding meridian and discussed accordingly. The meridians are also presented in the classical manner, beginning with the Meridian of the Heart. At the beginning of each section, you will find a short description of the meridian's course, its position in the circulation of energy, as well as its pulse position. Likewise, the points which belong to a meridian, but which are not located thereupon, in other words, the associated or concurring ("assentiment") points, and sometimes, alarm points, are also briefly noted. These are discussed in detail under the point's abbreviated name, in other words, all associated or concurring ("assentiment") points on the Meridian of the Bladder; possible alarm points, for example, that of the Heart Meridian, thus under CV 14.

The Conception and Pilot Vessels, which contain important points, are dealt with after the meridians.

The unit of the fingerbreadth (Chinese: CUN) always refers to the patient's finger, never to the physician's. Therefore, you must briefly study the form of the patient's fingers prior to treatment. This is very important, because otherwise, you will not be able to locate the point correctly.

THE MERIDIAN OF THE HEART

In general, we begin with this meridian. It receives its energy from the Meridian of the Spleen/Pancreas and passes it on to the Meridian of the Small Intestine. It is a YIN meridian. The abbreviation is H, in German as well; in French, C for coeur. Its pulse position is deep, distal to the radial apophysis on the left wrist. The meridian begins its course in the 3rd intercostal space on the anterior para-axillary line. Then, being a YIN meridian, it travels along the inner side of the upper extremity to the small finger, turns finally over to the dorsal side of the finger, and ends with its 9th point 2 mm medial and proximal to the corner of the cuticle. Its alarm point is CV 14, on the anterior midline about 1 fingerbreadth below the tip of the xiphoid. Its associated or concurring ("assentiment") point is B 15, on the back, about 2 fingerbreadths lateral to the midline between the transverse processes of the 5th and 6 th thoracic vertebrae (Fig. 4 and 6).

H 3

The first two points are not particularly significant. On the other hand, H 3 is an important point. Its Chinese name is **Shaohai**. Of course, it is not necessary to remember these names. I am only mentioning them because some authors include intersection points of one meridian or the other, or both, which might be confusing. If in doubt, comparison of the names will tell you immediately which point of our (most widespread!) numeration corresponds with the one described by another author. Exact translation of the names of the points is meaningless for us, and is therefore left out with only a few exceptions. However, some points also have an epithet which you should memorize for mnemonic purposes, such as H 3, which is called "Joy of Life." This epithet alone describes the indication. It is a point which is mainly acupunctured with a gold needle. It has a positive influence on the psyche. We use it as adjuvant in all disorders presenting negative psychological or depressive symptoms. It is also very effective for mental fatigue brought on by strong emotions. Again, I want to stress that endogenic depression, for example, is not suitable for routine acupuncture treatment. We know that the philosophy of acupuncture correlates the heart and the psyche, just as in our philosophy and proverbs, the

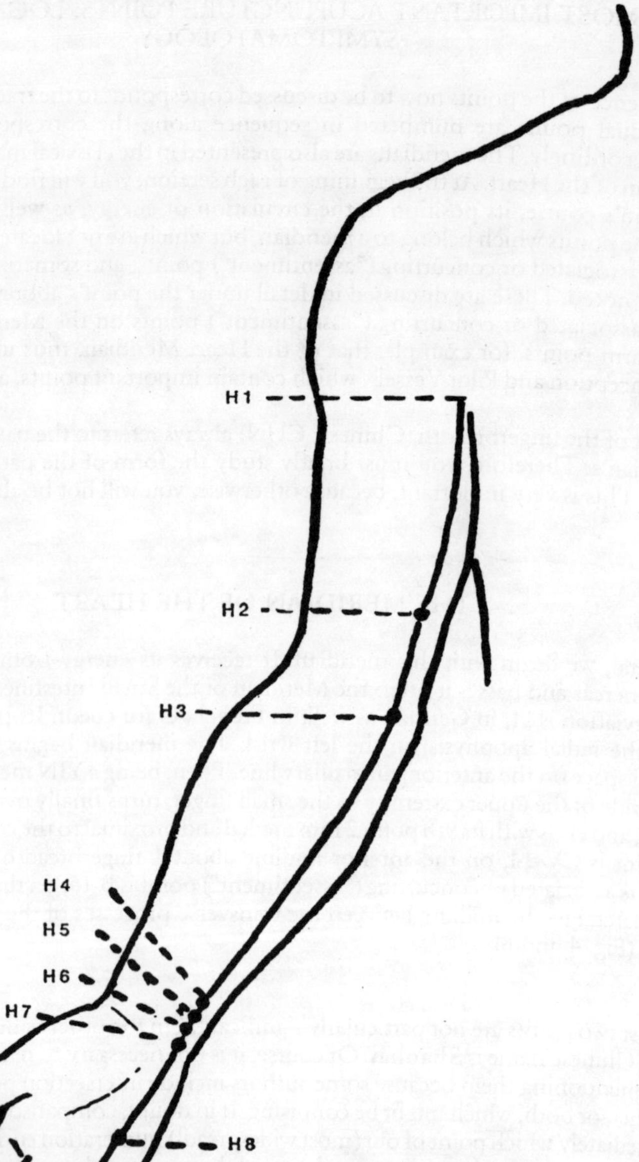

Fig 4

heart is not just seen as a pumping organ. Indications concerning the heart's mechanical or pumping action are: tendency to faint, increase in resistance, especially to infection, as well as palpitations following minimal exertion. Locally, it travelling along the upper extremity, the indications are: trembling hands (excluding *Parkinson's* disease), and cold and clammy fingers. *Location:* On the medial end of the fold of the elbow, which is formed when the elbow is bent as far as possible. It is easy to find and is often used.

H 5

Chinese name: **Tongli.** It is the passage or Lo point of the Meridian of the Heart, that means, it primarily represents the connection to its partner meridian, the Meridian of the Small Intestine. It enables us to balance varyingly strong Heart and Small Intestine pulses with only one needle. In such cases, you need not sedate or tonify the Heart and Small Intestine meridians individually. Indications: Here too, we have a strong psychological action, especially when combined with H 7 for stagefright, fear of examinations, and all types of nervous complaints of the heart. Locally, it helps influence paresis and spasms of the upper extremities. As a passage point it of course is (just as end or starting points of a meridian are) related to its partner organ as well. (The end or starting points to preceding or following meridians). Therefore, intestinal atonia and a hollow feeling in the stomach are also indications.
Location: Volar, over the ulnar artery on the level of the ulnar apophysis. Like all meridian points, it is found on both the left and right sides of the body in the same position (mirrored) and is hence always needled bilaterally.

H 7

Chinese name: **Shenmen.** This is both the sedation and source point of the Meridian of the Heart. Because the source point supports the sedation or tonification point, it can happen that, for example, both H 7 and H 9 are acupunctured with gold needles during the same session. However, because the body obviously possesses sufficient selective mechanisms, this presents no problems in an appropriate case. It also has a strong psychological action, especially when combined with H 5. Other indications are tachycardia with arrhythmia, anginose complaints, and the so-called angina pectoris. Here, we use it simultaneously as sedation point and sedating source point. However, it can also be used supportively as a tonifying source point when gold is used, for example in the treatment of hypotension (combined with other points), and bradycardia (together with H 9).
Location: On the radial side of the pisiform bone. The easiest way to find it is to palpate this region with a bellied bougie or the tip of a ballpoint pen. When indicated, it is always extremely painful upon pressure and the patient will show its exact location.

H 9

Chinese name: **Shaochong.** This is the meridian's tonification point. Main indications are bradycardia, circulatory weakness, and the so-called angina pectoris. If a patient faints during a treatment, or blacks out, and collapses (which usually only happens to robust men and does not mean that acupuncture is contra-indicated – indeed, this is sometimes accompanied by rapid and extensive improvement), H 9 and/or P 9 will immediately normalize his condition, whereby just massaging the point with the fingernail is often sufficient. Therefore, it is an important point for emergency acupuncture. As stated above, being end point of a meridian, it is also related to the next meridian (similar to a passage point), and is therefore also indicated for anorexia and slow digestion.
Location: About 2 mm medial and proximal to the cuticle of the small finger on its medial or thumb-side. The YIN meridian (which should always be on the inner side of an extremity) has turned to the dorsal, YANG side in its very last portion. Because the next meridian, which is its partner, is a YANG meridian (Small Intestine), it will also begin on the YANG (dorsal) side. It begins on the lateral side of the cuticle (just outside it) of the small finger. The connection of

these starting and end points is always via a so-called secondary vessel. Such secondary vessels are quite common in acupuncture, however, they are of little significance for the beginner.

THE MERIDIAN OF THE SMALL INTESTINE

As just described, this meridian receives its energy from the Meridian of the Heart and passes it on to the Meridian of the Bladder. The Small Intestine is a so-called YANG meridian. Its abbreviation is SI; in German, Dü for Dünndarm, and in French, IG for Intestine Grêle. Because its partner is the Meridian of the Heart, its pulse position is the same as that of the Heart (*left* wrist, distal to the radial apophysis), however, being a YANG meridian, its pulse point is in the *superficial* and *not* in the deep position. Being a YANG meridian, it travels along the outer side of the extremity from the outer corner of the cuticle of the small finger over the lower and upper arm laterodorsally to the shoulder where it forms an angle and then travels on along the lateral part of the neck to the cheek and from there, to its end point in the middle of the earlobe, all of this bilaterally of course. The Meridian of the Small Intestine has 19 points. Its alarm point is CV 4 (on the ventral midline, about 2 fingerbreadths above the symphysis). Its associated or concurring ("assentiment") point is B 27 (on the posterior superior iliac spine)

SI 1

Chinese name: **Shaoze.** This is the meridian's starting point. Because the Meridian of the Small Intestine has a strong affinity with all processes of the mucous membrane, we often use this point simply as adjuvant; hence not only for irritations of the intestinal mucous membrane, but for all treatments of catarrhal inflammations of the mucous membranes, including conjunctivitis, rhinitis, vaginitis, etc. You will already have noticed that the functional groups are often much more extensive in acupuncture than in our conventional medicine.
Location: 2 mm lateral and proximal to the cuticle of the small finger on the dorsal side.

SI 3

Chinese name: **Houxi.** This is the meridian's tonification point, and at the same time a cardinal point. That means it is a connection point for the "extraordinary vessels" or – using a short and poor translation – "wonder meridians". Use thereof requires more experience with acupuncture and pulse diagnosis, which is why they are purposely not discussed here. SI 3's main indication is spasmolysis. For this, it is usually combined with Li 2 and 3. Its second main field of importance is action – again in general – on all mucous membranes. As a tonification point it acts on atonic constipation, anorexia and (taking the psychological influence of the Meridian of the Heart into consideration) the depressive symptoms which accompany them. Likewise, it is also effective for paresis of the upper extremity, especially when the patient complains of sudden pain which radiates to the back. It is an important and frequently-used point.
Location: When the hand is closed in a fist, it lies on the lateral end of the skin fold behind (proximal to) the metacarpophalangeal joint of the small finger.

SI 4

Chinese name: **Wangu.** This is the meridian's source point. Therefore, its scope of action includes both indications requiring sedation and those requiring tonification. Aside from atonic intestinal disorders, it is especially effective for muscular weakness and lack of strength in the upper extremities; here, it is usually acupunctured with a gold needle. For spasms of the upper abdomen, diarrhea with colic, as well as spasms and arthritis of the hand and lower arm (especially writer's cramp), and also for "splitting" headaches correlated with menstruation, it is acupunctured with a silver needle.

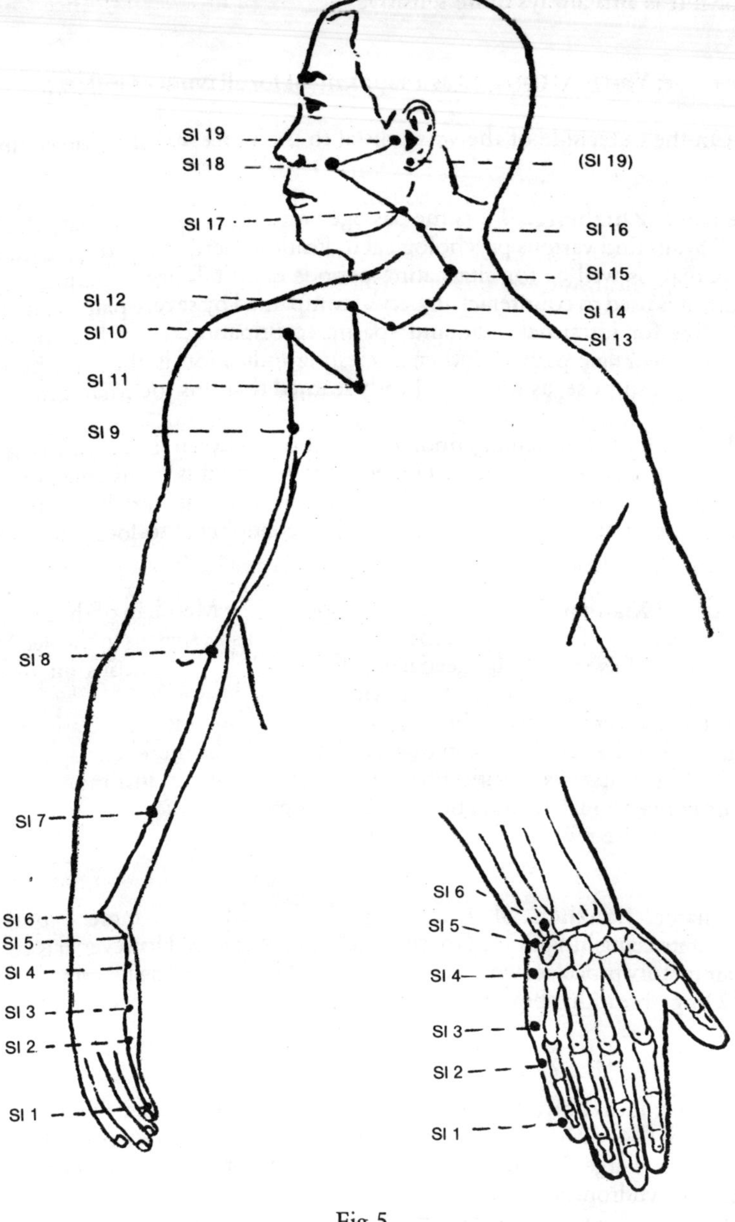
SI 19
SI 18
(SI 19)
SI 17
SI 16
SI 15
SI 12
SI 14
SI 10
SI 13
SI 11
SI 9
SI 8
SI 7
SI 6
SI 5
SI 4
SI 3
SI 2
SI 1
SI 6
SI 5
SI 4
SI 3
SI 2
SI 1

Fig 5

Location: On the lateral edge of the hand over the articulation of the 5th metacarpal and the hamate bone. It is also always quite sensitive.

SI 5

Chinese name: **Yanggu.** It is used as a supplement for all types of inflammation and pain in the hand.
Location: On the outer side of the wrist, distal to the processus styloideus ulnae.

SI 7

Chinese name: **Zhizheng.** SI 7 is the passage point to its partner organ, the Heart. Therefore, we will again find various psychological indications here. It is effective for neurasthenia, especially sexual, as well as for alternating periods of irritability and apathetic depression. Furthermore, it is used to counteract anxiety accompanied by severe palpitations. Of course, it is also effective for intestinal colic and spastic constipation, as well as purely locally for rheumatic and neuralgic pain. Another interesting indication is the stye, however, this no longer comes as a surprise, as we have already learned that this meridian acts on the mucous membrane.
Location: It is somewhat difficult to find, being halfway between the crease of the wrist and the elbow on the dorsal edge of the ulna. The best way to find it is to visualize the course of the meridian from SI 4 to 8. The point is in the middle of this imaginary line; a bougie or similar instrument, or an electric measuring device, may be employed to locate it exactly.

SI 8

Chinese name: **Xiaohai.** This is the sedation point of the Meridian of the Small Intestine. It is effective for all types of intestinal spasm, and also for muscle spasms in the neck or upper part of the back, as well as spasmodic headaches. In regard to the mucous membrane, it has a supportive action in the treatment of gingivitis.
Location: On the lower portion of the edge of the olecranon. It is used relatively infrequently. Again, you see that the so-called main or special points of the meridians do not always play a major role in the therapy of a specific disorder. However, they gain in importance when, on the basis of our conventional examinations and experience, the diagnosis is unclear and only palpation of the pulse reveals definite indications.

SI 9

Chinese name: **Jianzhen.** SI 9, for example, is used much more frequently than 8, irrespective of its being insignificant for the regulation of energy. However, it is very important for all inflammatory processes which prevent the patient from lifting his arm towards the back.
Location: 2 fingerbreadths above the dorsal end of the axillar fold when the arm hangs loosely to the side.

SI 15

Chinese name: **Jianzhongshu.** We now see for the first time a point of intersection of three meridans, in this case with 3H (point 16) and G (point 21). The point is also very close to the Meridian of the Large Intestine. It is mainly used for cervical migraine, cervical and cervicobrachial syndromes, as well as for spastic torticollis.
Location: On the outer side of the neck where, when viewed from the dorsal side, the trapezius muscle bends sharply laterally, that is, the medial beginning of the shoulder area.

SI 18

Chinese name: **Quanliao.** This point is frequently used for facial paralysis, trigeminal neuralgia and pain in the maxilla, as well as for trismus.
Location: On the anterior point of attachment of the masseter to the cheekbone in the angle formed from both.

SI 19

Chinese name: **Tinggong.** This point is used for weakness of vision, that is, for reduced visual acuity, but not for changes in the eyeball, such as in myopia etc. (By the way, an old method of improving eyesight – found in our folk medicine as well – was to wear a gold earring or the like on this spot!).
Location: In the middle of the earlobe, ventral, on the spot commonly pierced for earrings. New Chinese literature has moved this point away from the earlobe to the point of attachment of the auricle (approximately in the area of G 2). Recent Chinese data often contain new point locations. In crass cases, I will always point this out and add an explanation whenever possible, however, we do not consider these changes to be improvements or of particular significance.

That concludes the Meridian of the Small Intestine, or at least the most important points thereof.
The longest meridian having the most points is

THE MERIDIAN OF THE BLADDER

The Meridian of the Bladder receives its energy from the Small Intestine and passes it on to its partner organ, the Kidney. It is a YANG meridian and its pulse point is on the *left* wrist, proximal to the radial apophysis in the *superficial* position. Abbreviations: English and German: B; French: V (Vessie). It starts in the angle formed by the root of the nose and the corner of the orbit of the eye, travels latero-proximally over the head and then downwards about 2 fingerbreadths laterally to the dorsal midline until it reaches the sacral horn. Then it jumps back to the shoulder blade (having no points in this portion), or, what is more probable, it has a second branch 2 fingerbreadths farther lateral starting at the level of Th 1/2. This branch then descends dorsally over the back, buttocks, and behind the knee to the lower leg. In the middle of the lower leg, it curves to the lateral side and reaches the edge of the foot dorsal to the external malleolus, and then travels laterally to the lateral corner of the small toe, where it ends with its 67th point just outside the cuticle. All associated or concurring ("assentiment") points including its own, of course, lie on the first branch of this meridian, that is, the one which is closest to the posterior midline. Its alarm point. CV 3, is about 2 fingerbreadths above the symphysis on the anterior midline.

This meridian's main sphere of action is elimination. Let's begin with B 1 (Fig. 6).

B 1

Its Chinese name is **Jingming.** Here again we find indications from the preceding meridian, such as conjunctivitis, blepharitis, and especially sinusitis. It is also an important point for cephalaea, especially frontal headache.
Location: In the angle formed by the root of the nose and the orbit, approximately where the noserests of eyeglasses leave a mark. Many people rub this point instinctively when they have a headache.

B 2

Chinese name: **Zanzhu.** This is the main point for all headache and sinusitis treatments. Together with the single (that is, it has no partner) point PdM (Point de Merveille), which lies on the Pilot Vessel (PV) or **Tou-Mo,** it forms the so-called "triangle magique anterieur", or "frontal magic triangle". This emphasizes the almost "magical", rapid and lasting response in the above indications. It is a very important and frequently-used point.
Location: On the point of intersection of an imaginary perpendicular line through the nasal angle of the eyelid with the line of the eyebrow just above the supraorbital foramen.

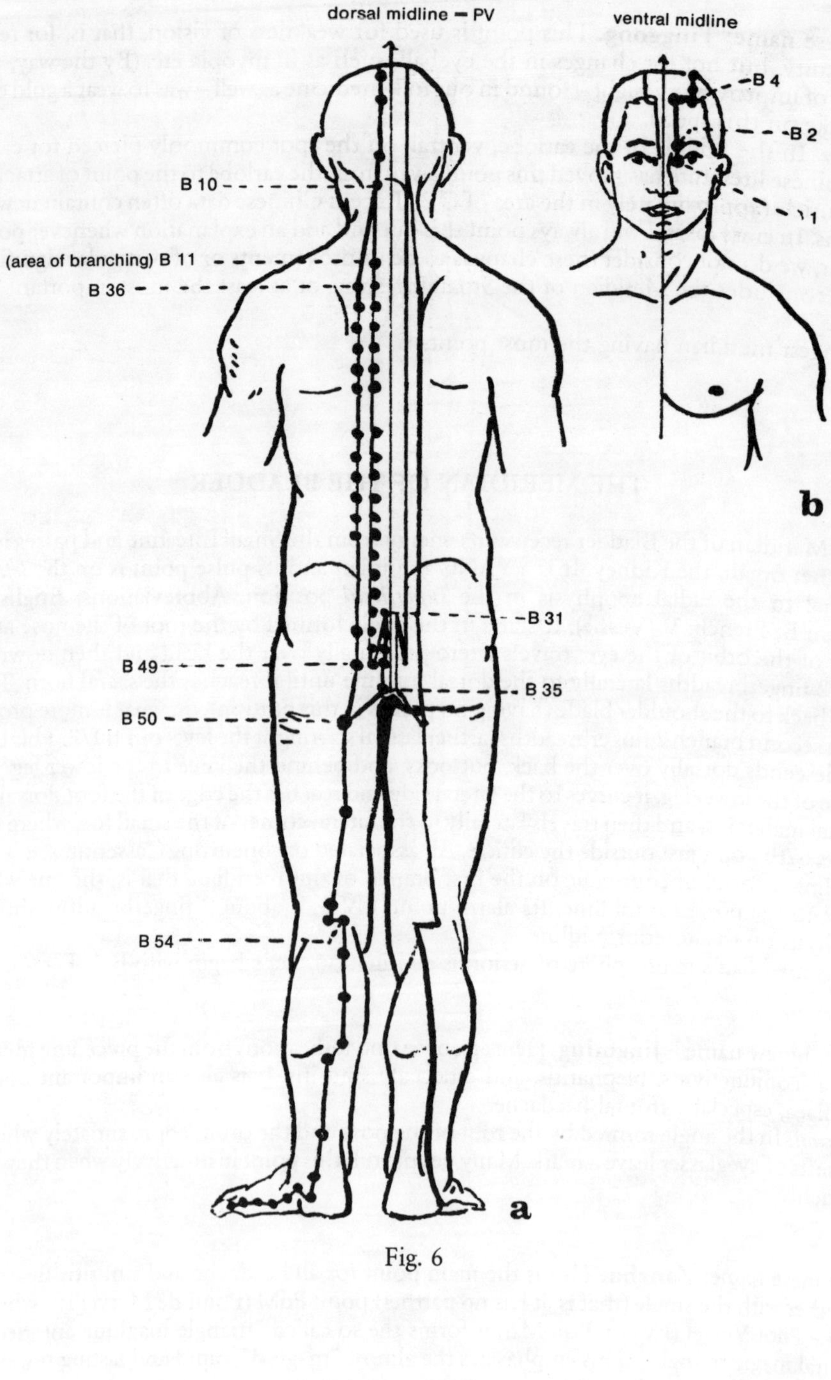
dorsal midline – PV
ventral midline
B 4
B 2
B 1
B 10
(area of branching) B 11
B 36
B 31
B 49
B 35
B 50
B 54
b
a

Fig. 6

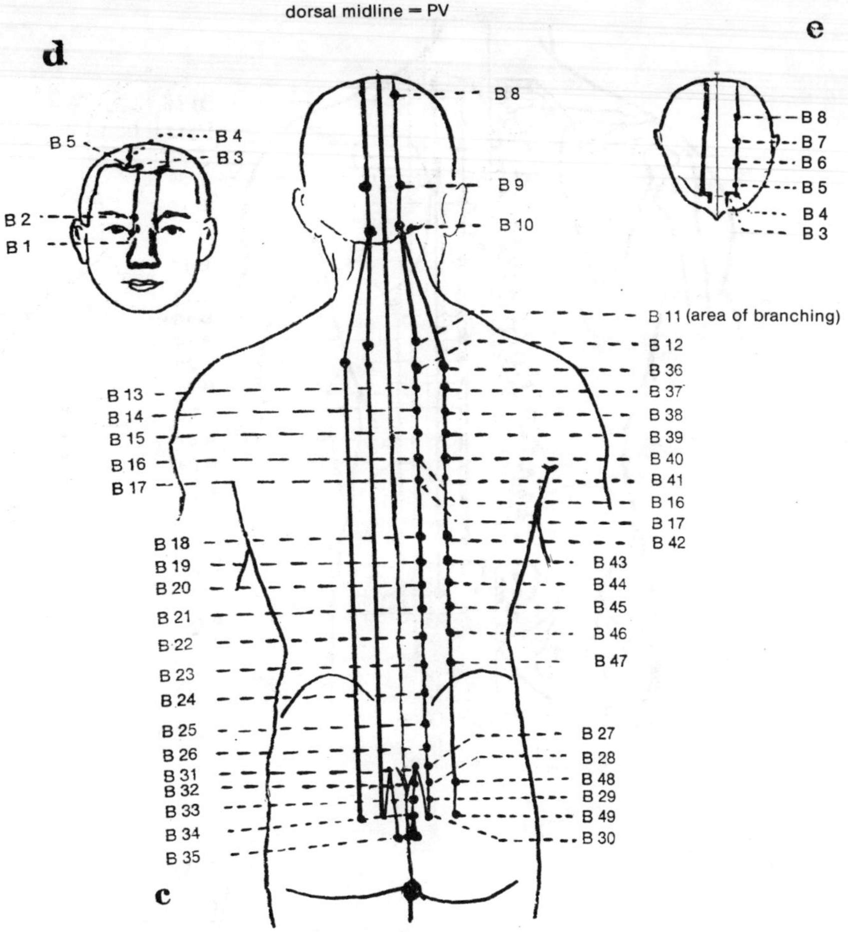
dorsal midline = PV
d
B 5
B 4
B 3
B 2
B 1
c
B 8
B 9
B 10
B 11 (area of branching)
B 12
B 36
B 37
B 38
B 39
B 40
B 41
B 16
B 17
B 42
B 13
B 14
B 15
B 16
B 17
B 18
B 19
B 20
B 21
B 22
B 23
B 24
B 25
B 26
B 31
B 32
B 33
B 34
B 35
B 43
B 44
B 45
B 46
B 47
B 27
B 28
B 48
B 29
B 49
B 30
e
B 8
B 7
B 6
B 5
B 4
B 3

Fig. 6

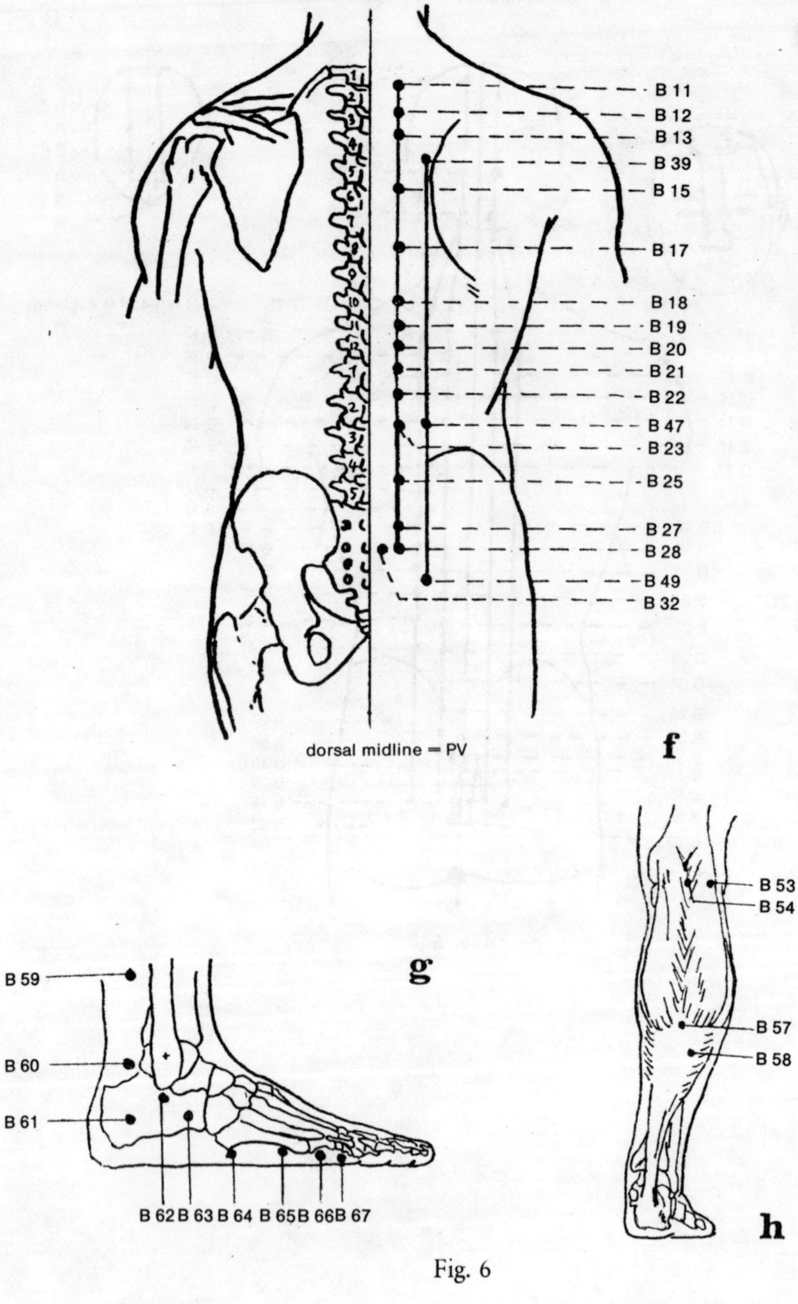
B 11
B 12
B 13
B 39
B 15
B 17
B 18
B 19
B 20
B 21
B 22
B 47
B 23
B 25
B 27
B 28
B 49
B 32
dorsal midline = PV
f
B 53
B 54
B 57
B 58
h
B 59
B 60
B 61
B 62
B 63
B 64
B 65
B 66
B 67
g

Fig. 6

B 4
Chinese name: **Quchai.** Mainly used as a supplementary point for frontal headache; less frequently for trigeminal neuralgia of the first branch and also for vertigo.
Location: Somewhat more than 2 fingerbreadths lateral to the midline, about 2 fingerbreadths above the hairline (or where it once was, which can usually be recognized by the different skin color).

B 8 (In new Chinese reports, this point is often called B 9)
Chinese name: **Luoque.** It lies on the tubera of the head on the level of the lambdoid suture, 2 fingerbreadths lateral to the midline. We use it as a supplementary point for headache and migraines, as well as for petit mal.

B 10
Chinese name: **Tianzhu.** This is another important acupuncture point. Generally speaking, it has a strong effect on the nose and eye, that means particularly sinusitis and inflammatory affections of the eye and nose. Furthermore, when combined with B 1 and/or 2, it has a strong influence on all forms of cephalaea. It seems to generally stimulate the blood circulation in the head. The point is also important for the treatment of anosmia. It is also effective for all types of cervical syndrome. Indeed, this type of pain almost always radiates to the lower occipital region exactly to this point. Last but not least, it has a general effect on the vagus. Thus, it can also lower blood pressure and may be included in the specific treatment program for all vagotonic disorders. Hence, it is a very important point!
Location: This point is found on the lower edge of the squama occipitalis, 2 fingerbreadths lateral to the dorsal midline. All the subsequent points down to B 27 are also found at this distance from the midline.

B 11
Chinese name: **Dazhu.** This point is important locally; besides, it is an adjuvant in the treatment of bone diseases. Spontaneous sensitivity or sensibility to pressure on this point alone can be considered an indication of the presence of a bone disorder, without, however, giving any information as to the site of the process (together with G 30).
Location: Again 2 fingerbreadths lateral to the dorsal midline, this time between the transverse processes of the 1st and 2nd thoracic vertebrae. In describing all of the subsequent points, I shall only give the number of the vertebrae between the transverse processes of which each point is found.

B 12
Chinese name: **Fengmen.** This point is found in the regular course of the Meridian of the Bladder, between Th 2 and 3. It is a supportive point for the treatment of asthma and bronchitis and is also often effective for sinusitis.

B 13
Chinese name: **Feishu.** This is the first associated or concurring ("assentiment") point we come to. It is the associated (concurring) point of the Lung. To review briefly: An associated or concurring ("assentiment") point always lies on the (first branch of the) Meridian of the Bladder regardless to which meridian it belongs. Associated (concurring) points are always used when no significant progress is being made with a well-selected (according to the pulse) treatment program for a chronic disorder. These points can be acupunctured with gold or silver needles. Sometimes, especially when they are spontaneously sensitive, they can also be administered right at the beginning of a treatment. Their Chinese name always ends with "shu". B 13 is used for bronchitis, dyspnea, dry cough, and especially bronchial asthma.
Location: Between the 3rd and 4th thoracic vertebrae.

B 14

Chinese name: **Jueyinshu.** This is the associated (concurring) point of the Pericardium or Envelope of the Heart. It is used particularly for chronic disorders of the circulatory system and sexual organs.
Location: Between the 4th and 5th thoracic vertebrae.

B 15

Chinese name: **Xinshu.** This is the associated (concurring) point of the Meridian of the Heart. It is used relatively often, especially for stagefright and mental depression, almost always combined with H 3, 5, and 7; it is used less frequently as a supplementary point for writer's cramp, tremor, and vertigo; of course, also for the various sensations of the heart such as tachycardia and bradycardia.
Location: Between the 5th and 6th thoracic vertebrae.

B 17

Chinese name: **Geshu.** This is a very important point. It is not an associated (concurring) point of an organ meridian, but has a pronounced effect on the diaphragm's range of movement, as well as on all types of circulatory disorders. It is also effective in the treatment of diseases of the blood, particularly influencing the venous components, to which end it is usually used together with SP 5 and K 8. We use this point mainly for *Roemheld's* syndrome, for the treatment of bronchial asthma, angina pectoris, especially the so-called angine pectorale fausse and also for the regulation of blood coagulation. *Bergsmann* also uses this point as adjuvant in the treatment of pulmonary tuberculosis and was the first to demonstrate both spirometrically and by x-ray that this point has a prompt action on the diaphragm and hence, achieves a significant increase in breathing capacity. The use of this point can sometimes lead to syncope, especially when the needle is inserted somewhat deeper in unstable individuals. This complication is counteracted with H 9 or P 9.
Location: Between the 7th and 8th thoracic vertebrae.

B 18

Chinese name: **Ganshu.** This is the associated (concurring) point of the Liver and is used for all types of liver disorders and often for stomach disorders as well.
Location: Between the 9th and 10th thoracic vertebrae.

B 19

Chinese name: **Danshu.** Associated (concurring) point of the Meridian of the Gallbladder. It is used supplementarily for all diseases of the gallbladder. Children who vomit after drinking milk represent a less common indication for this point.
Location: Between the 10th and 11th thoracic vertebrae.

B 20

Chinese name: **Pishu.** This is the associated (concurring) point of the Meridian of the Spleen-Pancreas. It is used for general digestive disorders, usually combined with B 18, 19, and 21. It is rarely used alone, usually only as a supplement in the treatment of anemia.
Location: Between the 11th and 12th thoracic vertebrae.

B 21

Chinese name: **Weishu.** Associated (concurring) point of the Stomach. It is also called "the Master Point of the Stomach". This expression implies a point's special characteristics. It is also effective for all stomach disorders ranging from ulcers to gastritis. Furthermore, it has a distinct effect on stomach cramps including pylorospasm and is often used against singultus. It is used very frequently, as stomach disorders respond well to acupuncture treatment.

Location: Between the 12th thoracic and 1st lumbar vertebrae.

B 22
Chinese name: **Sanjiaoshu.** This is the associated (concurring) point of the Meridian of the Triple Heater (3H). It is used quite rarely; actually only as a supplement for all types of disorders of the respiratory, digestive, and urogenital tracts.
Location: Between the 1st and 2nd lumbar vertebrae.

B 23
Chinese name: **Shenshu.** Associated (concurring) point of the Meridian of the Kidney. Because the Chinese regard the adrenal gland and the kidneys as a unit, we find fatigue and weariness as the main indications. It also has a strong action on all rheumatic conditions – usually combined with 3H 5. We also like to use B 23 against diarrhea, when the influential factor of worsening due to cold is significant. As already mentioned, the kidney is the organ least accessible to acupuncture, and therefore, the point is relatively rarely used for the treatment of chronic inflammations of the kidney and bladder.
Location: Between the 2nd and 3rd lumbar vertebrae.

B 25
Chinese name: **Dachangshu.** B 25 is the associated (concurring) point of the Large Intestine. It is mainly used for all types of constipation.
Location: Between the 4th and 5th lumbar vertebrae.

B 27
Chinese name: **Xiachangshu.** This is the associated (concurring) point of the Small Intestine. It is used particularly against diarrhea, usually together with SP 4. However, this point is often reverted to for all types of intestinal colic. Incidentally, it is also effective in the treatment of cystitis.
Location: On the posterior superior iliac spine.

B 28
Chinese name: **Pangguangshu.** Associated (concurring) point of the Meridian of the Bladder. It is used for all types of disorders of the urinary tract, and especially as a supplementary point in the treatment of sciatica and lumbago.
Location: Here, we leave the foregoing line of associated (concurring) points to find this point 3 fingerbreadths lateral to the lower edge of the second sacral foramen.

B 31
Chinese name: **Shangliao.** This is a very important point. We also call it "the Master Point of Climacterium". It has a strong hormonal action in women, not only during menopause, especially when combined with 3H 22 and SP 6. This point should be used at least once during an acupuncture treatment on women around the age of 50 regardless of the actual reason treatment is being given. As if that were not enough, it is also one of the most important points for the therapy of sciatica and lumbago especially when the patient complains of cold extremities. It is one of acupuncture's most important and most frequently-used points, again, without being the main point of a meridian.
Location: In the distal, medial quadrant of the first sacral foramen.

B 33
Chinese name: **Zhongliao.** As is B 34, B 33 is combined with B 31, especially for the so-called high sciatic neuritis.
Location: B 33 lies in the 3rd sacral foramen in the same position as B 31 in the first.

B 34

Chinese name: **Xialiao** (according to *Bachmann* and the latest reports from China). It lies on the inner side of the gluteal fold on the level of the sacral horn. It has a supportive action on some types of sciatica and on "connective tissue weakness".

The meridian now curves upwards as described above, that is, the numeration of the points of the second branch commences in the scapular area. All points after B 36 are located 4 fingerbreadths lateral to the dorsal midline.

B 39 (also called B 38 in many books)

Chinese name: **Gaohuang.** This is an important, generally tonifying point. Use of this point may also cause the patient to collapse. It is used against anemia, general weakness, reduced resistance, especially in convalescence; also as an adjuvant in the treatment of bronchitis. It also has a sedating action, hence, is indicated especially for singultus (hiccoughs), as well as for spasms and neuralgia in the upper thoracic region and the shoulders.
Location: It is somewhat difficult to find. The best method is to have the patient sit with his knees together and bend over arching his back. Now, B 39, which is on the point of intersection of the scapula and the upper edge of the fourth rib, becomes accessible. In normal posture, it is covered by the scapula.

B 47

Chinese name: **Zhishi.** This point is often used for badly itching dermatoses and all chronic skin diseases. However, it is also used quite often as a supplementary point in the treatment of rheumatism.
Location: This point lies 1 fingerbreadth above the iliac crest and 4 fingerbreadths lateral to the dorsal midline on the point of intersection of the two. It is always sensitive to pressure.

B 50

Chinese name: **Chengfu.** B 50 is an important point for the therapy of sciatica.
Location: In the middle of the gluteal fold. It is identical to the *Valleix* pressure point with which we are familiar.

B 54

Chinese name: **Weizhong.** This is a very important point and also a so-called metabolic point. Therefore, it has a strong influence on skin diseases. Letting this point bleed a little is advisable. Furthermore, it is a very important point for the treatment of paresis of the lower extremities. In these cases, the needle is inserted somewhat deeper. It is mainly acupunctured with a gold needle for all these indications. For the treatment of sciatica and all spastic processes in the lower extremity, especially osteoarthritis of the knee, it is acupunctured with a silver needle. This point as well is used often; in almost every case.
Location: When the knee is bent, as in a sitting position, B 54 lies in the middle of the popliteal space. If the patient is standing or has his leg stretched out, it lies about 1 fingerbreadth thereabove, however, always on the midline.

B 58

Chinese name: **Feiyang.** This is the Lo or passage point of the Meridian of the Bladder, and establishes the connection to the partner Meridian of the Kidney. It is also a metabolic point and thus has a general action on metabolic disturbances. One of its main indications is intermittent claudication, however, it is also effective for any other spastic or painful process in the entire lower extremity. Therefore, it plays just as important a role in therapy of sciatica as in the treatment of paresis. It should be acupunctured in every case of osteoarthritis of the knee and included in any treatment of the ankle or foot. As already mentioned, it is extremely important that in cases of painful or inflammatory conditions limited to individual joints, the

adjacent joints (proximal and distal) also be included in the treatment. Finally, we must not lose sight of the fact that we are approaching the end of the meridian, and that in difficult cases, the initial portion of the meridian can and must be influenced therefrom (and vice-versa!). Thus we often use B 58 (usually combined with B 60, 64, 65, and 67) in the treatment of cephalaea.
Location: This point lies on the lateral side of the calf above the soleus muscle on the level of the angle formed by the caput tibialis and the caput fibulae of the musculus gastrocnemius. It is easy to find, at least easier than the description might lead you to believe. This is a very important acupuncture point.

B 60

Chinese name: **Kunlun.** This too is a very important point. It is the so-called Master Point of all Pain, that means, pain can be basically influenced by this point regardless of where in the body it is felt. It is used particularly in the treatment of sciatica, but also for all muscle cramps in the lower extremity, as well as the long erector muscles of the back. Furthermore, it is very effective for the treatment of edema of the ankle if the edema is not caused by a cardiac disorder. Therefore, especially after removal of casts, an amazingly fast reduction of swelling may be observed.
Location: This point is found on the upper, lateral border of the calcaneum in the middle of an imaginary line between the external malleolus and Achilles tendon.

B 62

Chinese name: **Shenmai.** This is another cardinal point. Its main action is against insomnia, used together with K 6. However, it is also indicated for other manifestations of nervous agitation, especially those in which the influential factor of worsening during menstruation is important. We also use this point for spastic and atonic paresis or complaints in the lower extremities, of course also for swelling of the ankles. You can also try using it for resistant headaches.
Location: This point is found 2 fingerbreadths below the distal tip of the external malleolus, where the change in pigment of the tissue begins. It is easy to find and is an important point.

B 64

Chinese name: **Jinggu.** This is the meridian's source point. Therefore, it has many indications, of YANG as well as YIN. It is acupunctured with gold or silver needles depending on the individual indications, which range from depression with refusal to eat, splitting headaches, neuralgia, and cramps in the legs, to cervical syndrome and blepharitis, just to name the most important. It is used frequently, especially for headache.
Location: B 64 lies on the outer edge of the foot proximal to the capitulum of the fifth metarsal bone.

B 65

Chinese name: **Shugu.** B 65 is a sedation point. We use it especially for cramps in the calf, sciatica, and "crawling ants" in the legs. It often proves to be very effective in the treatment of acne (together with several metabolic points).
Location: Also on the outer edge of the foot, just proximal to the metatarsophalangeal joint of the fifth toe.

B 67

Chinese name: **Zhiyin.** B 67 is the tonification point. It is mainly used for emotional excitation, but also for exhaustion, hypotension and a "worn-out feeling". It can be used to facilitate and promote childbirth, an advantage for doctors in rural areas. It is also effective for frontal headache and conjunctivitis.

Location: Similar to SI 1, it lies 2 mm proximal and lateral to the outer corner of the cuticle of the fifth toe. Acupuncture of this point is quite painful.

Now, we have completed the discussion of this long meridian and can begin with

THE MERIDIAN OF THE KIDNEY

The Meridian of the Kidney receives its energy from the Meridian of the Bladder and passes it on to the Meridian of the Pericardium (or Envelope of the Heart). It is a YIN meridian. Abbreviations: English: K; German: N (Niere); French: R (Rein). Its pulse point is found on the *left* wrist, just like that of the Bladder, proximal to the radial apophysis but in the *deep* position. The meridian begins on the sole of the foot, in-between the aspects of the first and fifth metatarsophalangeal joints (where bunions form), then, as a YIN meridian, turns to the inner side of the foot, travels over the leg and groin, being the meridian closest to the midline, then ventrally upwards on the torso, and ends with its 27th point on the lower border of the sternoclavicular joint. Its alarm point is the point G 25 on the free end of the 12th rib. Its associated (concurring) point is B 23 (Fig. 7).

K 1

Chinese name: **Yonquan.** It is the first sedation point (there can be several sedation and alarm points). Its most important indications are absence of, or insufficient perspiration, mental indecision, flatulent dyspepsia, and cystitis. It is also occasionally used as adjuvant in the treatment of asthma.

Location: As described above, on the sole of the foot between the aspects of the first and fifth metatarsophalangeal joints. Because acupuncture of this point is quite painful, the patient tends to jerk backwards when needled, thus, the best method is to insert the needle while the patient is kneeling on a chair (if you use this point at all, which will not be too often).

K 2

Chinese name: **Rangu.** K 2 is the second sedation point. Nevertheless, some of its indications are the complete opposite of those of K 1, for example, excessive perspiration and exaggerated tendency to make decisions. It, too, is used for cystitis, and acne as well, as it is also a metabolic point. Furthermore, we use this point for swollen ankles, rheumatic complaints of the lower extremities, especially for "burning feet" during the night; less frequently for bronchitis and pharyngitis.

Location: On the medial side of the foot, just below the protrusion of the navicular bone.

K 3

Chinese name: **Taixi.** Here, the Chinese names become practical for the first time. In his standard work, "Die Akupunktur – eine Ordnungstherapie" (Ulm, 1959, Karl F. Haug Publishers), *Bachmann* simplified the course of the meridian somewhat; at any rate, he changed it. For us (and in all other books), K 3 is identical to the point he calls K 5. All points after K 7 are again congruent. Therefore, please watch for discrepancies in some books with respect to these five points.

Be it as it may, this point is the source point. We mainly use it together with K 7 (gold) for severe, general fatigue. When silver is used, a distinct change is frequently achieved via this point, especially in the treatment of rheumatism. It is used less frequently as an additional point for bronchial asthma and angina pectoris.

Location: Half a fingerbreadth below and behind the internal malleolus.

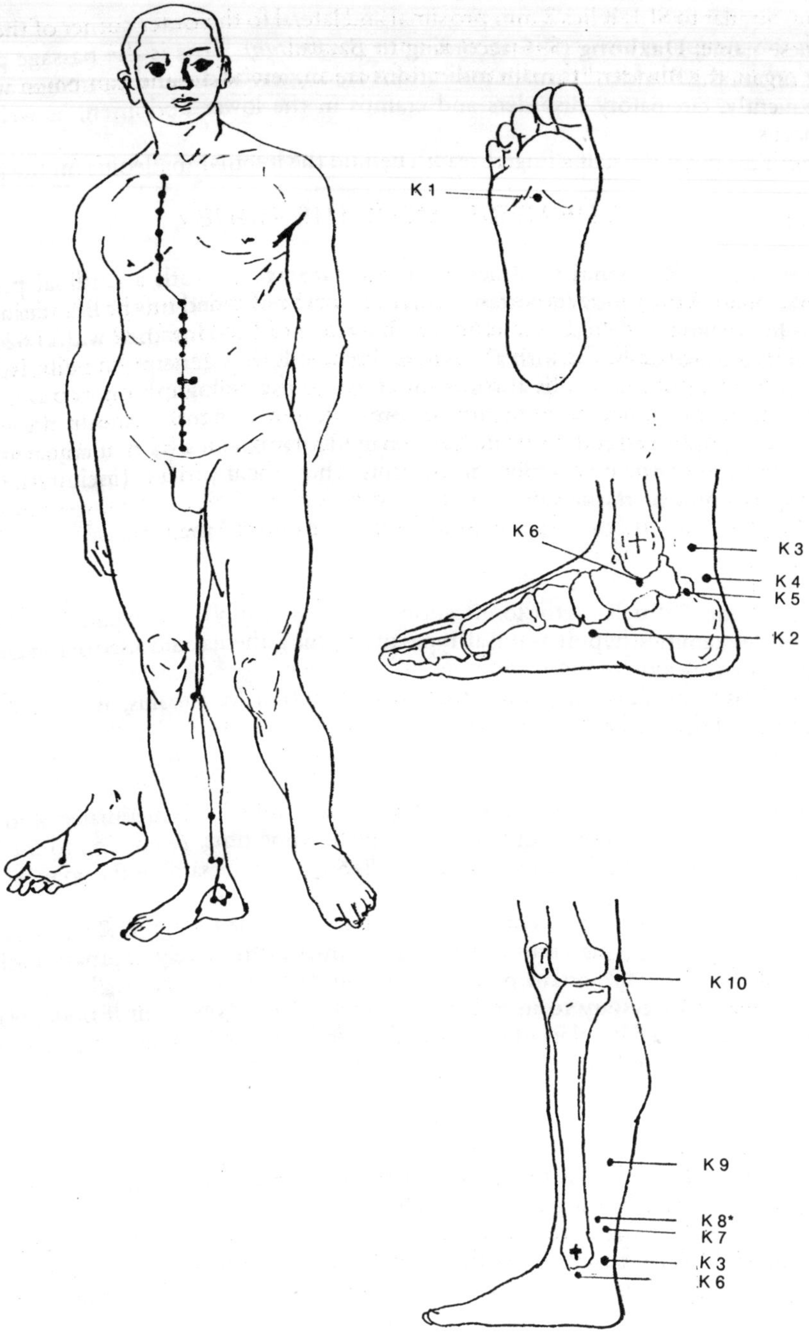

*Point of intersection or area of approximation

Fig. 7

K 4

Chinese name: **Dazhong** (K 6 according to *Bachmann)*. This is the passage point to its partner organ, the Bladder. Its main indications are anxiety and sadness, tremor and vertigo; less frequently, circulatory disorders and cramps in the lower abdomen, as well as in the oesophagus.
Location: This point lies half a fingerbreadth behind the internal malleolus on the level of the tip thereof.

K 6

Chinese name: **Zhaochai** (K 3 according to *Bachmann)*. Both a cardinal point and a metabolic point, hence, very important. I have already mentioned this point, stating that it is effective for insomnia when acupunctured with a gold needle, combined with B 62 (silver). If both points are acupunctured with a silver needle, they have a general pain-alleviative effect, similar to B 60. However, K 6 is also a main point for psychological tonification, especially when the influential factor of worsening in connection with menstruation is present. It also facilitates uncomplicated childbirth and is often used for migraines, particularly in women, for which its positive, regulative action on the entire hormonal process (including menstrual disorders, etc.) may be responsible.
Location: This point lies one fingerbreadth below the internal malleolus.

K 7

Chinese name: **Fuliu.** K 7 is the tonification point. It is mainly used for paresis and weakness of the lower extremities, hypotension, all types of psychic asthenia, and also for hot flashes, less frequently for adnexitis.
Location: This point lies 3 fingerbreadths above the internal malleolus, about half a fingerbreadth behind the medial edge of the tibia.

K 8

Chinese name: **Jiaoxin.** "The intersection of the three YIN meridians of the lower extremity". It is also the points Li 5 and SP 6 at the same time. According to *Bachmann's* nomenclature, this point is SP 6. The point he calls K 8 is not the same as the point we are now discussing.

It is well known that this point would be better described as SP 6. This is not a real intersection, but rather, the locus at which the 3 meridians closely approach each other. Because this is a very important point (for acupuncture analgesia as well as acupuncture therapy), I find it necessary to introduce it to you already now, even if under a perhaps improper name. Since SP is the last meridian discussed, and this point is significant for many already-mentioned combinations, I find this exchange completely justified for learning purposes.

K 8 is a very important acupuncture point. Being a point of intersection, it has several completely different indications. Another epithet for this point is "Master of the Blood." In fact, it has a regulative action on the blood supply of the entire lower extremity all the way up to the small pelvis, making it just as effective for all menstrual disturbances (hence, hyper as well as hypofunction) as for hyper and hypotension. Furthermore, it is effective against diarrhea and constipation and spasms and pain in the entire leg and hip. We also use its (here, probably mainly hormonal) action for mental agitation. Don't let the extent and seeming contradiction of the indications scare you. As you already know, acupuncture is primarily a regulative therapy and, therefore, always has a balancing and normalizing effect. That is what differentiates it from our conventional medicine, which always tries to accost a disorder as directly as possible, and only very rarely consciously addresses the body's own regulative powers.
Location: This point lies 4 fingerbreadths above the tip of the internal malleolus on the medial edge of the tibia and is always distinctly sensitive.

K 11

Chinese name: **Henggu.** This is the second alarm point of the Pericardium (or Envelope of the Heart) Meridian. Its main indications are impotence and frigidity, conditions of deficient or excessive sexual excitation, as are those of the subsequent points of the Meridian of the Kidney.

Location: On the upper edge of the pubis, 1 fingerbreadth lateral to the symphysis.

K 13

Chinese names (for this point, there are three): **Qixue, Baomen, Zihu.** It lies 3 fingerbreadths – sometimes higher, up to 4 fingerbreadths – above the upper edge of the pubis, 2½ fingerbreadths lateral to the ventral midline. It is helpful for meno and metrorrhagia as well as for constipation and general weakness.

K 14

Chinese name: **Siman.** This point has the same indications as 13 and 15 is located between the two. All these points are mainly of interest when the extraordinary vessel, TCHRONG-MO, is used. The beginner rarely needs them.

K 15

Chinese name: **Zhongzhu.** See above for indications. It lies approximately on the point of intersection of an imaginary line 2½ fingerbreadths lateral to the ventral midline; about one fingerbreadth below the navel.

K 21

Chinese Name: **Youmen.** The effectiveness of this point is mainly revealed in the treatment of hyperemesis gravidarum and (together with B 39) singultus (hiccoughs).

Location: On the tip of the angle between the 6th and 7th costal cartilage on the level of the 6th intercostal space.

All the subsequent points of the Meridian of the Kidney have the same location, each one intercostal space above the other (with the exception of the 3rd) and are of some significance as adjuvants in the therapy of bronchial asthma.

K 27

Chinese name: **Shufu.** This is one of the most important points for the treatment of asthma. An influential factor also indicating use thereof is worsening from cold and dampness. However, this point has another special characteristic. While all meridian points are basically acupunctured bilaterally, this point may on occasion be acupunctured on the left side only for psychasthenia or similar conditions.

Location: On the edge of the sternum, on the lower part of the sternoclavicular joint.

This concludes the Meridian of the Kidney and, at the same time, the first cycle of energy. That means that the energy was transported centrifugally from the lateral side of the thorax to the fingers (in the Meridian of the Heart) and from there centripetally via the Meridian of the Small Intestine to the head, and then centrifugally over the torso to the toes in the course of the Meridian of the Bladder, and, finally returned centripetally from there to the thorax via the Meridian of the Kidney, the discussion of which has just been completed.

This cycle is repeated twice beginning with

THE PERICARDIUM (ENVELOPE OF THE HEART) MERIDIAN

This meridian receives its energy from the Meridian of the Kidney and passes it on to the Meridian of the Triple Heater. This is a YIN meridian. We abbreviate it as P. In French, it is termed Maitre du Coeur, MdC, or Enveloppe du Coeur et Sexualité, ECS; in German it is also called „Meister des Herzens" (Master of the Heart); the abbreviation is KS („Kreislauf-Sexualität"). Its pulse position is on the *right* wrist, proximal to the radial apophysis in the *deep* position. The meridian begins in the 4th intercostal space, one fingerbreadth lateral to the mammilla and travels downwards from there along the inner side of the upper and lower arm to the middle of the volar crease of the wrist, and ends, similar to the Meridian of the Heart, by finally turning to the dorsal side 2 mm medial and proximal to the corner of the cuticle of the middle finger. Its associated or concurring ("assentiment") point is B 14; its second alarm point is K 11; the first alarm point is P 1 (Fig. 8).

P 1

Chinese name: **Tianchi.** As first alarm point, it is effective for angina pectoris, palpitations of the heart and as a supplement in the treatment of hyper and hypotension.
Location: In the 4th intercostal space, one fingerbreadth lateral to the mammilla.

P 6

Chinese name: **Neiguan.** This very important point is both the cardinal point and the passage or Lo point of this meridian to its partner meridian, the Triple Heater. Its main significance is as a regulative point for circulation in general, hence, also of blood pressure, and therefore, it is often used in the treatment of all types of cephalaea, especially migraines. This is largely due to the fact of its also having an extensive action on hormonal and sexual functions. It is also often used for all types of psychasthenia. In addition, when the needle is inserted deeper, it has a long-lasting effect on all types of paresis of the upper extremities. In China it was the main point used in the treatment of malaria.
Location: P 6 lies on the anterior midline of the lower arm, 3 fingerbreadths above (proximal to) the middle of the largest crease of the wrist.

P 7

Chinese name: **Daling.** P 7 is both sedation and source point. It has circulatory, hormonal, and sexual effects very similar to P 6, and can also be alternated with the latter. It also plays a significant role in the treatment of intercostal neuralgia and writer's cramp, as well as herpes zoster.
Location: In the middle of the largest volar crease of the wrist.

P 9

Chinese name: **Zhongchong.** This is the tonification point. Its main function has already been described: It counteracts syncope, not only during the acupuncture treatment itself. It is also effective for hypotension, congestion (in the brain), and even sexual dysfunction and menstrual disorders (very generally speaking). It has also proven to be effective locally for numbness of the hands and neuralgic pain in the arms.
Location: 2 mm medial and proximal to the medial corner of the cuticle of the middle finger (thumb side) after the meridian has turned to the dorsal side (like the Meridian of the Heart).

This concludes the discussion of this meridian which consists of two functions. We now come to the meridian which seems the strangest to us,

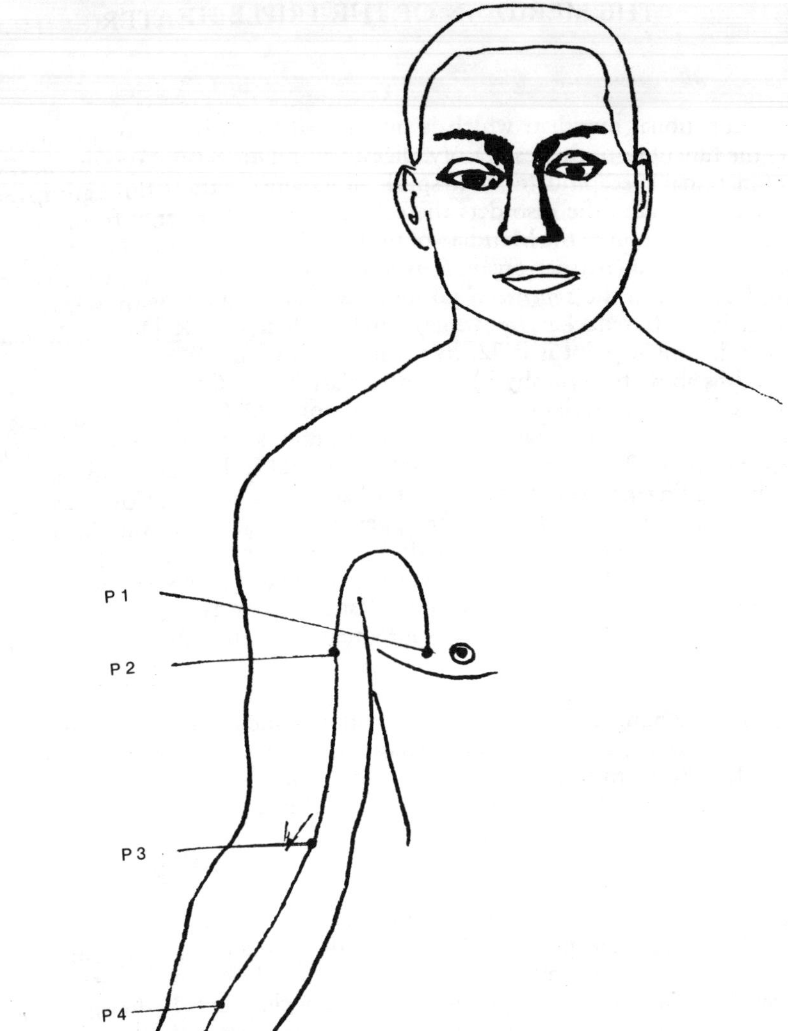

Fig. 8

THE MERIDIAN OF THE TRIPLE HEATER

This is a functional meridian which is not related to an organ of its own, but rather, comprises the functions of the respiratory, digestive, and urogenital systems in their entirety. Hence, it functionally recapitulates, so to speak, all activities of these three groups and its list of indications also includes the disorders thereof. It receives its energy from the Pericardium Meridian and passes it on to the Meridian of the Gallbladder. It is a YANG meridian. Its pulse position, like that of its partner organ, P, is found on the *right* wrist proximal to the radial apophysis, however, in the *superficial* position. We abbreviate it with 3H. In German, the abbreviation is 3E (Dreifacher Erwärmer); in French it is TrR (Triple Réchauffeur). Its associated (concurring) point is B 22; its main alarm point, CV 5 (on the ventral midline, 3 fingerbreadths above the symphysis); its sexual alarm point, CV 7 (one fingerbreadth below the navel); its digestive (simultaneously that of the stomach), CV 12 (a good 2 fingerbreadths below the xiphoid), and its respiratory, CV 17 (in the middle of the sternum on the level of the 4th intercostal space). The meridian begins 2 mm lateral and proximal to the corner of the cuticle of the ring finger, travels dorsally over the back of the hand and lower arm to the elbow, and then, travelling dorsolaterally over the upper arm, it reaches the middle of the shoulder. From there it travels over the lateral part of the neck to the ventral side of the mastoid process, circles the ear and ends in the indentation between the tragus and the attachment of the auricle. Newer Chinese data presents the course of the last portion as being somewhat different (see points 21-23). The first two points are less important than the subsequent ones (Fig. 9).

3H 3

Chinese name: **Zhangzhu.** 3H 3 is the tonification point. It is important for the treatment of congestive headache, arthritis of the fingers and joints of the hand; for psychological and sexual disorders. Furthermore, it is able to provide lasting help in convalescence.
Location: On the back of the hand in the angle formed proximal to the 4th and 5th metacarpals.

3H 4

Chinese name: **Yangchi.** 3H 4 is the meridian's source point. Aside from indications of a sexual and genital nature, its main significance is as the master point for vasomotor headache. Simple massage of this point with the fingernail is often sufficient to alleviate such headaches immediately, thus enabling prognostically important conclusions to be drawn. Secondly, it has a lasting effect, for example, after removal of a cast, on weakness of the hand after fractures, as well as in cases of paralysis. These two indications render this point very important.
Location: 3H 4 lies on the back of the hand over the articulation between the hamate bone and the 4th metacarpal. The easiest way to locate it is to move the fingernail of your slightly bent index finger proximally over the dorsal side of the 4th metacarpal using slight pressure until the nail actually falls into the articulation. There, one feels the tendons, on the medial side of which the point lies. It is painful when palpated with the fingernail and cannot be overlooked.

3H 5

Chinese name: **Waiguan.** A very important point! It is the cardinal point and Lo, or passage, point to the partner organ, Pericardium. It is our main point for general treatment of rheumatism. Therefore, it must not be omitted from any treatment of rheumatism. Furthermore, it is also effective for all types of paresis of the upper extremities and all types of headache, especially those which worsen when the weather changes. Together with LI 4, it is also very effective for all types of burning eczema. Hence, like most cardinal points, it has a very broad spectrum.

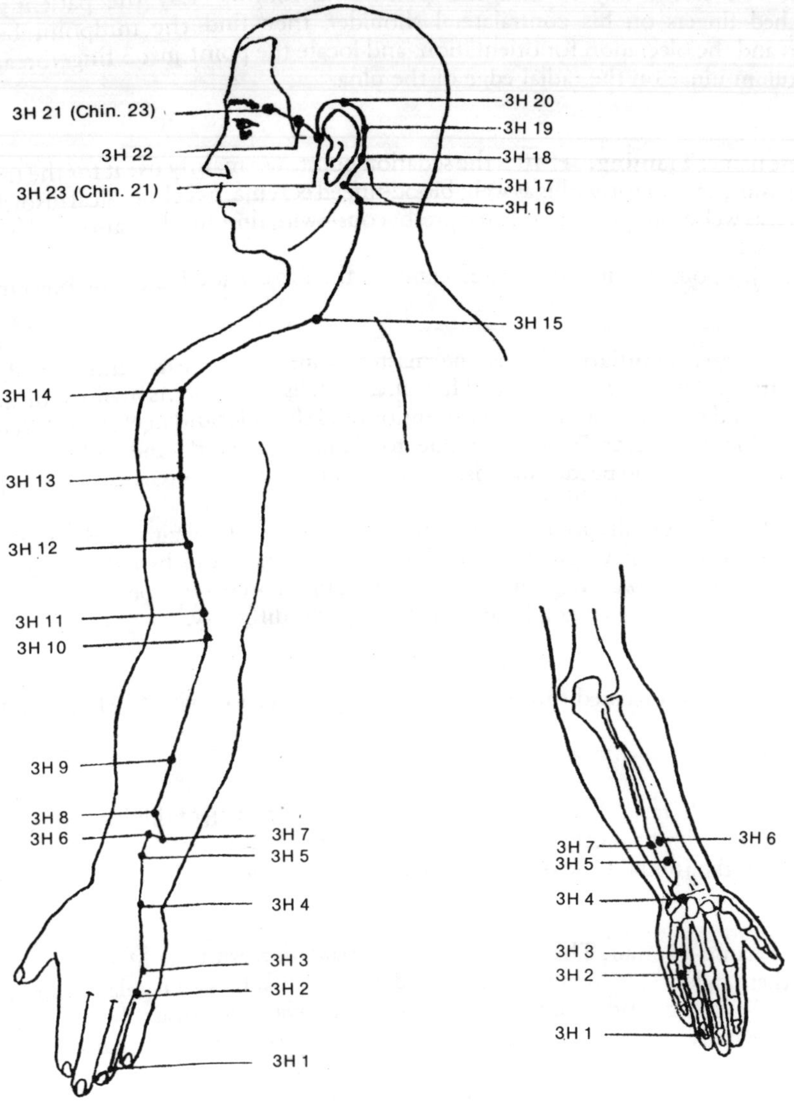
3H 21 (Chin. 23)
3H 22
3H 23 (Chin. 21)
3H 20
3H 19
3H 18
3H 17
3H 16
3H 15
3H 14
3H 13
3H 12
3H 11
3H 10
3H 9
3H 8
3H 6
3H 7
3H 5
3H 4
3H 3
3H 2
3H 1
3H 6
3H 7
3H 5
3H 4
3H 3
3H 2
3H 1

Fig. 9

Location: The easiest way to find this point is as follows: Lay the patient's arm with outstretched fingers on his contralateral shoulder, then find the midpoint between the fingertips and the olecranon for orientation, and locate the point just 3 fingerbreadths above the capitulum ulnae on the radial edge of the ulna.

3H 10

Chinese name: **Tianjing.** 3H 10 is the sedation point. We mainly use it for the treatment of muscle spasms, and for torticollis as well; blood-tinged eczema, psychological disorders caused by anxiety, as well as supplementarily for presbycousis with tinnitus. It is also used occasionally for headache.
Location: This point lies in the fossa olecrani on the proximal edge of the olecranon itself.

3H 15

Chinese name: **Tianliao.** This is the master point of the arms and was also named "hygrometric point" by *De la Fuye.* That already tells us what its main indications are: rheumatism and neuralgia of the upper extremities and shoulder and neck, as well as torticollis. For the influential factor "worsening due to dampness, wind, and cold", it is usually acupunctured with a gold needle; likewise for paresis of the arms. Thus, another very important point for daily practice on this meridian.
Location: 3H 15 is usually found on the upper edge of the trapezius in the middle of the shoulder, however, it may sometimes be located 1-2 fingerbreadths below and somewhat lateral to that locus. However, because it is so painful upon pressure, especially in persons who are sensitive to weather changes, locating it presents no difficulty.

3H 16

We have already discussed this point as point of intersection with G 21 and SI 15 in the section on the latter.

3H 17

Chinese name: **Yifeng.** This point is important in the treatment of rhinitis and sinusitis, and often, tinnitus. It immediately eases breathing through the nose.
Location: On the frontal edge of the mastoid behind the lobe of the ear.

3H 22

Chinese name: **Heliao.** This is the point of intersection with the Meridian of the Gallbladder, there called G 3 and usually used under that name. It has a regulative action on the blood supply in the head. Therefore, it is used particularly for headache, once again, for migraines, as it also has a strong effect on the female genitals and hormonal factors. Via this point, menstruation can be inhibited (you should always make young women aware of this fact prior to treatment!), and therefore, it should not be acupunctured during the first three days of menstruation. Acupuncture of this point, too, may lead to syncope. We also use it for rhinitis. It is a very important point.
Location: Half a fingerbreadth above the middle of the cheek bone.

3H 23

Chinese name: **Ermen,** "the Gate to the Ear." Here for once the Chinese name really tells us about the point. It is the master point for any process in the ear, for example, tinnitus in particular, some types of hearing defects, otitis, and inflammations of the external auditory canal. In addition, it is important for treatment of facial paralysis, trigeminal neuralgia, sometimes for tics and trismus. An important point!

In recent Chinese articles, 3H 23 is called 3H 21. According thereto, 3H 23 lies just dorsal to G 1.

Location: In the indentation between the tragus and the upper point of attachment of the auricle.

THE MERIDIAN OF THE GALLBLADDER

The Meridian of the Gallbladder receives its energy from the Meridian of the Triple Heater and passes it on to the Meridian of the Liver. This is a YANG meridian. Abbreviations: English and German: G; French: Vb (Vesicule biliaire). Its pulse point is found on the *left* wrist directly over the radial apophysis in the *superficial* position. Its associated (concurring) point is B 19. The meridian begins in the angle formed by the orbital edge and the cheek bone, travels in several bizarre curves back and forth four times across the lateral side of the head, then reaches the dorsal portion of the mastoid, travels over the lateral part of the neck to the frontal axillary line. Then, its course approaches ever more closely the lateral line of the trunk down to the vertex of the iliac crest, which it follows ventrally, then crosses to the greater trochanter and travels on strictly laterally to the head of the fibula, then along the frontal edge of the fibula to the dorsum pedis, ending 2 mm proximal and lateral to the corner of the cuticle of the fourth toe. Several very important points lie on this meridian. Let us begin with (Fig. 10 and 11)

G 1

Chinese name: **Tongziliao.** Used for migraines and sinusitis together with G 2. As the most important point for ophthalmic disorders, it is used especially for conjunctivitis.
Location: In the angle orbital curve – cheek bone.

G 2

Chinese name: **Tinghui.** This is the more important of the two points. It is mainly used for ophthalmic migraine and is one of the standard points for the therapy of tinnitus.
Location: G 2 lies just in front of the lower point of attachment of the auricle on the level of the incisura intertragica.

G 3

Chinese name: **Shangguan.** This point has already been dealt with as 3H 22.

G 8

Chinese name: **Shuaigu.** About one fingerbreadth above the tip of the auricle and 2 fingerbreadths dorsal to this line. Its indications are the same as those of G 17; in addition, sinusitis, and less frequently torticollis.

G 14

Chinese name: **Yangbei.** This is the test point for gallbladder disorders in the presence of which it is particularly sensitive. Colics can be alleviated via this point. Furthermore, it is effective for frontal headache, trigeminal neuralgia of the first branch, tics, and conjunctivitis.
Location: Draw an imaginary perpendicular line through the middle of the pupil; the point lies 2 fingerbreadths above the eyebrow.

G 17

Chinese name: **Zhenying.** G 17 lies about 3 fingerbreadths lateral to the midline of the skull above the highest point of the auricle. It is used for headache and tinnitus.

G 19

Chinese name: **Naokong.** Supplementary point for treatment of tinnitus.

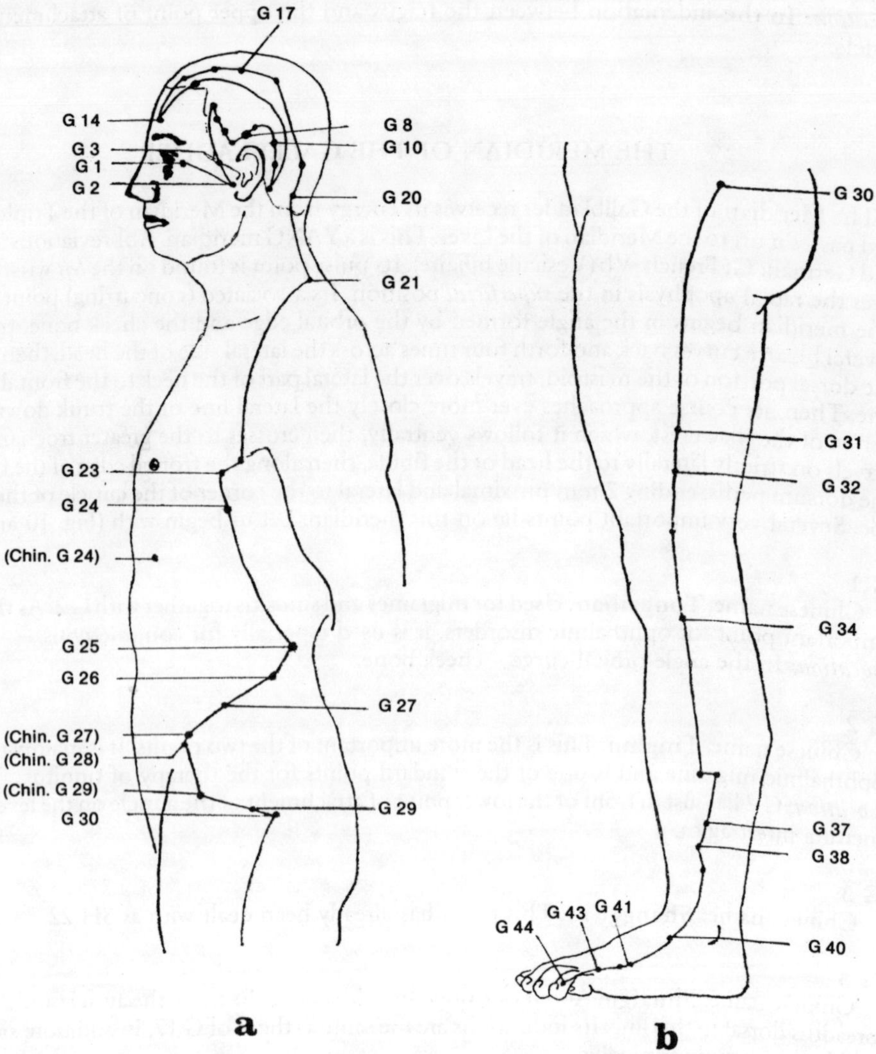
G 17
G 14
G 3
G 1
G 2
G 8
G 10
G 20
G 21
G 23
G 24
(Chin. G 24)
G 25
G 26
G 27
(Chin. G 27)
(Chin. G 28)
(Chin. G 29)
G 30
G 29
a
G 30
G 31
G 32
G 34
G 37
G 38
G 44
G 43
G 41
G 40
b

Fig. 10

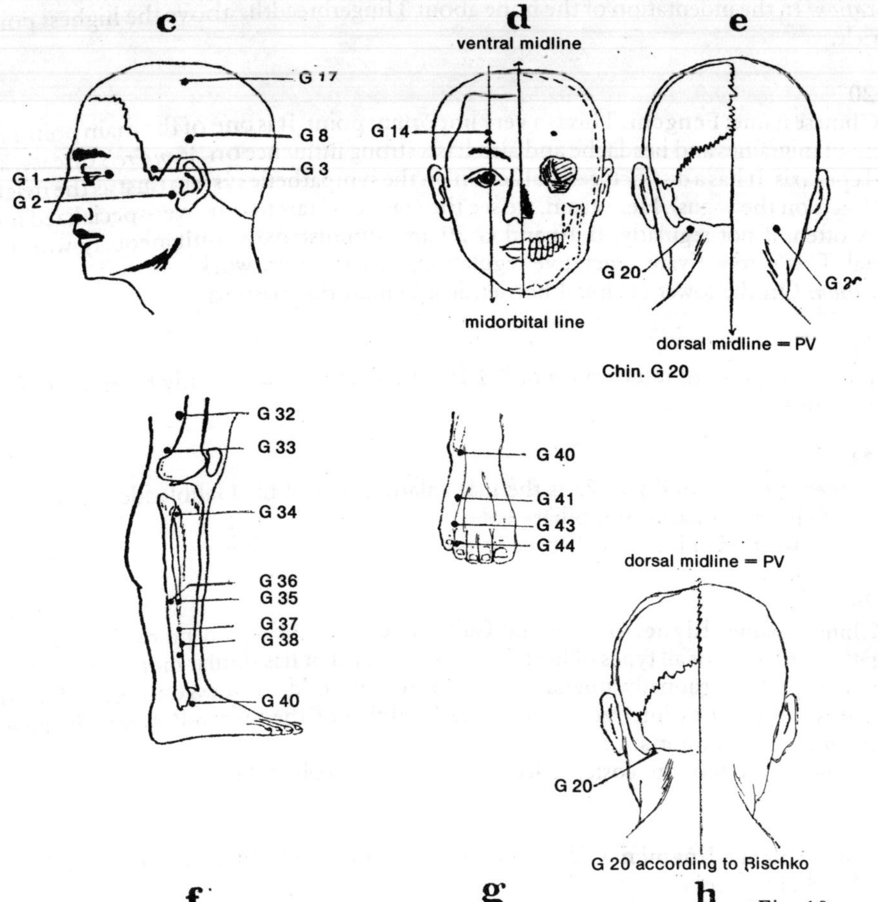
c
d
e
ventral midline
G 17
G 8
G 3
G 1
G 2
G 14
G 20
G 20
midorbital line
dorsal midline = PV
Chin. G 20
G 32
G 33
G 34
G 36
G 35
G 37
G 38
G 40
G 40
G 41
G 43
G 44
dorsal midline = PV
G 20
G 20 according to Bischko
f
g
h

Fig. 10

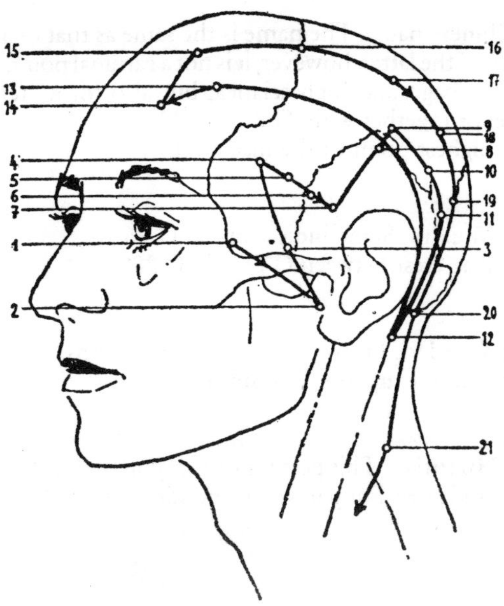
15
13
14
4
5
6
7
1
2
16
17
9
18
8
10
19
11
3
20
12
21

Fig. 11

Location: In the indentation of the bone about 3 fingerbreadths above the highest point of the auricle.

G 20

Chinese name: **Fengchi.** This is a very important point. It is one of the main points for treatment of migraines and headache and also has a strong influence on *Menière's* disease, sinusitis, and epistaxis. It has a distinct, general action on the sympathetic system (just as the neighboring B 10 acts on the vagus). Here again, we see the crass contrast to our over-specialized medicine. Very often, if not regularly, B 10 and G 20 are administered simultaneously with the same metal. This is to activate vegetative regulation, and as a rule, works.
Location: On the lower occipital border, just behind the mastoid.

G 21

This is the point of intersection of 3H 16 and SI 15 and has already been discussed under those terms.

G 23

Chinese name: **Zhejin.** G 23 is the main alarm point of the Gallbladder. It is used for all types of cholecystopathy and biliary colic.
Location: In the 5th intercostal space in the anterior axillary line.

G 24

Chinese name: **Riyue.** G 24 is the Gallbladder's second alarm point. It is mainly used together with Li 6 for all types of liver disorders; by itself, it has similar indications to G 23 plus flatulence and, occasionally, migraines. For the indication "drowsiness during the day", the fact that it is the point of intersection with the Meridian of the Spleen-Pancreas, it there being number 21, is of importance.
Location: In the 6th intercostal space on the anterior axillary line.

G 25

Chinese name: **Jingmen.** G 25 is the alarm point of the Kidney. It is used as adjuvant for renal and biliary colic.
Location: On the free end the 12th rib.

G 26

Daimai is its Chinese name. The name is the same as that of an "extraordinary meridian", and it is also a point of the latter, however, it is not a cardinal point. It is very important not only for treatment of lumbago and high sciatica, but also for all female genital and hormonal disorders, just like, or together with, G 27 and 28.
Location: On the highest point of the iliac crest.

G 27

Chinese name: **Wushu.** Same indications as G 26.
Location: On the iliac crest between G 26 and G 28.

G 28

Chinese name: **Weidao.** Likewise, the same indications.
Location: On the anterior superior iliac spine.

G 30

Chinese name: **Huantiao.** This point is very important for the therapy of sciatica, as well as arthritis of the hip and knee. For paresis, the needle is inserted deeply into this point. It is also

effective for skin rashes. Spontaneous pain on this point indicates the presence of a bone disorder, similar to B 11.
Location: G 30 is found on the most prominent point of the greater trochanter. If the patient is standing, or has his leg completely outstretched, it is located somewhat farther dorsally.

G 32
Chinese name: **Zhongdu.** A supplementary point for the therapy of sciatica.
Location: On the midpoint of an imaginary line connecting G 30 and G 34.

G 34
Chinese name: **Yanglingguan.** A very important point. It is called "the Master Point of the Musculature." Thus, we find it extremely valuable for all types of paralysis (of all muscles), as well as for pain and spasms. It also has a mild action on the blood circulation of the lower extremities and can also be used in the treatment of atonic constipation.
Location: In the indentation in front of and below the head of the fibula.

G 37
Chinese name: **Guangming.** G 37 is the meridian's passage or Lo point to its partner organ, the Liver. It is mainly used for biliary colics and all types of cholecystopathy, but also for neuralgia and paresthesia of the lower extremities, usually needled together with its immediate neighbor, G 38.
Location: G 37's position is somewhat complicated; on the lateral side of the leg, 3 fingerbreadths below the midpoint between the upper border of the tibia and the external malleolus.

G 38
Chinese name: **Yangfu.** G 38 is the sedation point. Its indications are the same as those of G 37; in addition, migrating pain in the entire body.
Location: 5 fingerbreadths above the tip of the external malleolus on the frontal edge of the fibula just below G 37.

G 40
Chinese name: **Qiuxu.** G 40 is the source point. It is effective for all types of spasms – abdominal and in the extremities – as well as for general weakness and fatigue.
Location: It is difficult to find; above the calcaneo-cuboid joint.

G 41
Chinese name: **Lingqi.** G 41 is a cardinal point and is very effective for all joint disorders, especially those of the large joints.
Location: Dorsal, in the angle formed by the 4th and 5th metatarsal bones.

G 43
Chinese name: **Xiaxi.** G 43 is the tonification point. It is mainly used for atonic constipation, sensation of fullness; less frequently for paresis of the legs; sometimes for inflammations of the eye and jaw, as well as for mastitis.
Location: On the lateral side of the metatarsophalangeal joint of the 4th toe, over the joint cavity.

THE MERIDIAN OF THE LIVER

The Meridian of the Liver receives its energy from the Meridian of the Gallbladder and passes it on to the Meridian of the Lung. It is a YIN meridian. Abbreviations: English: Li; German: Le (Leber); French: F (Foie). Its associated (concurring) point is B 18. Its pulse point is on the *left* wrist directly on the radial apophysis, however, this time in the *deep* position. The meridian starts 2 mm lateral and proximal to the corner of the cuticle of the big toe, then travels over the dorsal surface of the foot and along the medial side of the leg and thigh, continuing over the abdomen to the free end of the 11th rib and ending in the 5th intercostal space on the mammillary line (Fig. 12).

Li 2

Chinese name: **Xingjian.** Li 2 is the meridian's sedation point. This point is mainly important because of its strong spasmolytic action. It is usually used to promote spasmolysis together with Li 3. It is also an effective supplement for congestion and dysmenorrhea. Because of its spasmolytic action it is used frequently.
Location: On the lateral end of the joint cavity of the metatarsophalangeal joint of the large toe, that is, between the 1st and 2nd toes.

Li 3

Chinese name: **Taichong.** This is the source point. Its indications are practically the same as those of Li 2 plus paralyses in the tibial region. It is used particularly for all types of disorders afflicting the big toe.
Location: It is found in the proximal angle formed by the 1st and 2nd metatarsal bones.

Li 5a

Li 5a is synonymous with the points K 8 and SP 6 and has already been discussed.

Li 5

Chinese name: **Ligou.** Li 5 is the passage point to its partner organ, the Gallbladder. It is a frequently-used point because of the general importance of the liver. It is used particularly for general complaints, itching of the skin, and mild liver insufficiency. It is also effective for intestinal spasms and dysfunctions of the inner genital organs.
Location: On the medial edge of the tibia, 2 fingerbreadths below the midpoint between the upper edge of the tibia and the internal malleolus.

Li 9 (I would completely agree with calling this point Li 8, as is done in almost all other works. The different names are a result of divergencies in continuing numeration following points of intersection, and are therefore of negligible significance).

Chinese name: **Ququan.** Li 9 is the tonification point. It is frequently used because of its general action. It strengthens the body in general, physically as well as mentally. Therefore, it also has a whole list of conditions of vegetative, mental, and sexual weakness as indications, as well as spasms in the lower extremities, migrating pain, and stomach ulcers. Most important, however, is always its general, wide-range effect. We like to use it several times in the course of every treatment.
Location: On the medial end of the crease of the knee joint when it is maximally bent, or on the posterior, medial side of the knee joint cavity.

Li 12

Chinese name: **Jimai.** Frequently used for circulatory disorders of the legs; less frequently for dyspepsia and ophthalmic migraine.
Location: In the distal angle of *Scarpa's* triangle.

Li 13

Chinese name: **Zhangmen.** Li 13 is the alarm point of the Meridian of the Spleen-Pancreas. It is also a metabolic point. It is always used to combat general fatigue, in convalescence, as well

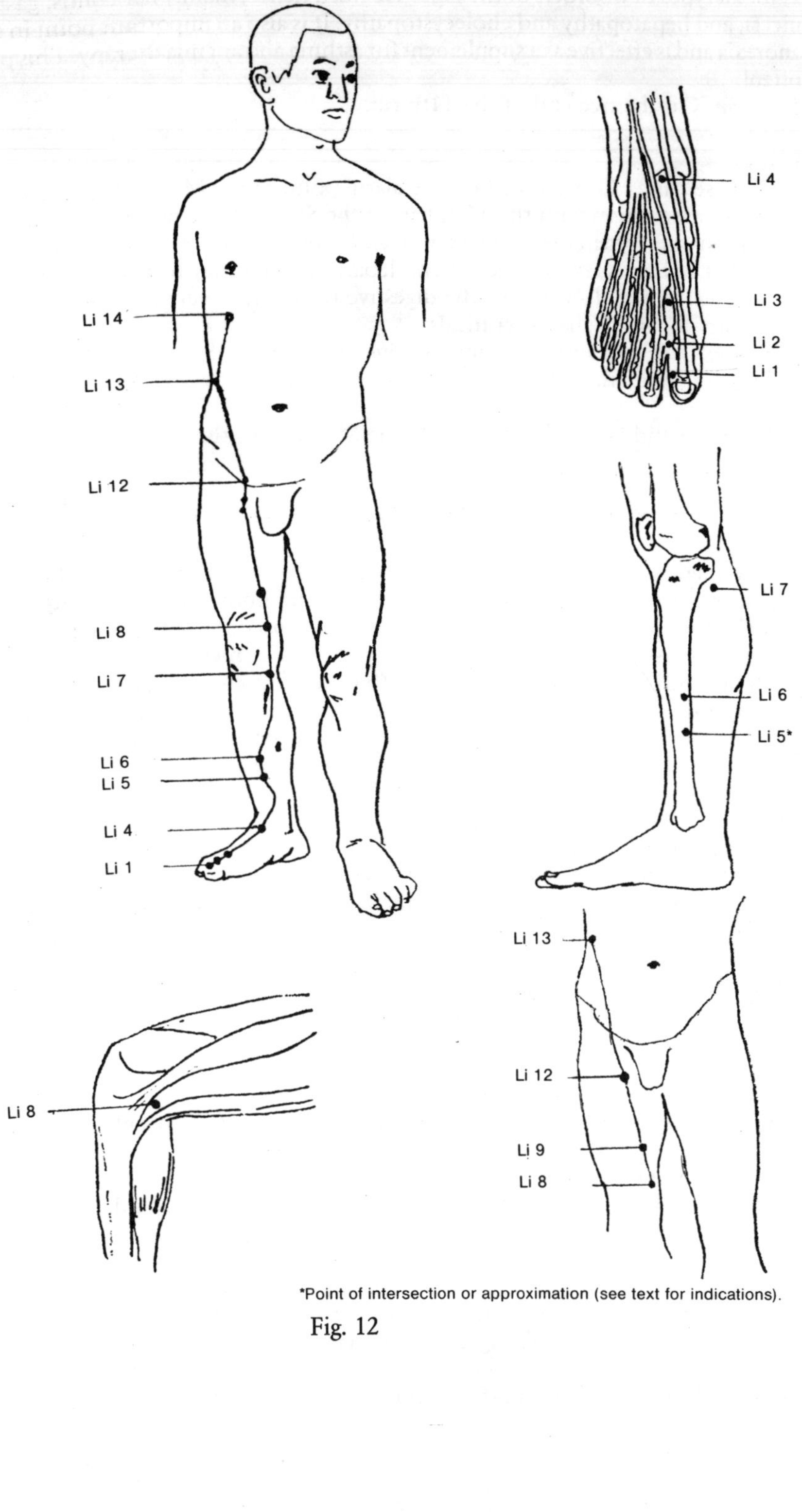

*Point of intersection or approximation (see text for indications).

Fig. 12

as for all types of disorders of the digestive tract, hence, mainly for colitis, gastritis, all types of ulcers, and hepatopathy and cholecystopathy. It is also an important point in the treatment of anorexia and is effective as a supplement for asthma and anemia therapy. This point is used very often!
Location: On the free end of the 11th rib.

Li 14

Chinese name: **Qimen.** Li 14 is the alarm point of the Meridian of the Liver and also the point of intersection with the Meridian of the Stomach, being number 18 thereof. Its main indications are: hyperemesis gravidarum and sea-sickness. For the latter, it is used preventively in the last few weeks before the patient departs on a journey by ship. It is very reliable. Other areas of usage are: disorders of the digestive tract with severe meteorism or flatulence. Less frequently for headaches after meals.
Location: On the mammillary line on the level of the 6th intercostal space.

That concludes the second cycle of energy. We have now arrived again at the lateral side of the chest.

The third and last cycle begins with the Meridian of the Lung.

THE MERIDIAN OF THE LUNG

This meridian receives its energy from the Meridian of the Liver and passes it on to the Meridian of the Large Intestine. It is a YIN meridian. Abbreviations: English and German: Lu; French: P (Poumon). Its pulse point is on the *right* wrist distal to the radial apophysis in the *deep* position. Its associated (concurring) point is B 13. The meridian starts on the frontal axillary line in the 3rd intercostal space, ascends to the 2nd intercostal space, and then travels to the anterior side of the upper arm. From there it continues downward along the forearm to the radial groove whereupon it circles the thumb and ends on the dorsal side thereof 2 mm lateral and proximal to the corner of the cuticle on the index finger side (Fig. 13).

Lu 1

Chinese name: **Zhongfu.** Lu 1 is the meridian's alarm point and at the same time a main point for treatment of all types of pulmonary disorders, especially asthma, usually together with Lu 2, B 13 and 17; K 27 and St 13. It is used less frequently for itching dermatoses.
Location: On the frontal axillary line on the level of the 3rd intercostal space.

Lu 2

Chinese name: **Yunmen.** Another main asthma point.
Location: Same as Lu 1, but in the 2nd intercostal space.

Lu 5

Chinese name: **Chize.** Lu 5 is the sedation point. It is mainly used for all types of dermatologic disorders in the face and also as a supplement in the treatment of spasms of the upper extremities, and asthma.
Location: In the middle of the crease of the elbow on the lateral border of the biceps tendon.

Lu 7

Chinese name: **Lieque.** Lu 7 is the passage or Lo point to its partner organ, the Large Intestine, and a cardinal point at the same time. However, it is mainly used as a main point in the treatment of all types of congestion. Furthermore, it is often employed as a remote point for asthma therapy and for headache, and also for all types of spasm and pain in the face (facial or trigeminal nerves) and hands. If the hemicrania is always on the same side, it is acupunctured

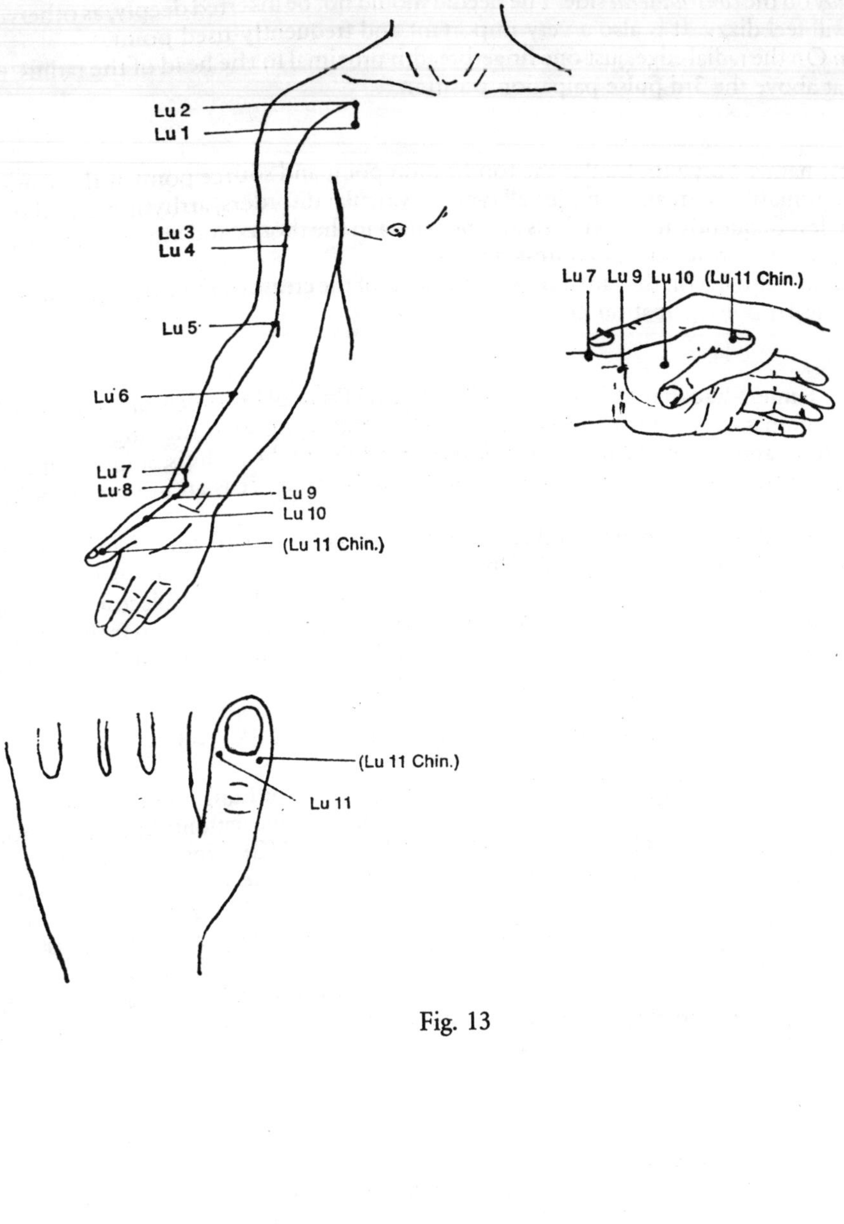
Lu 2
Lu 1
Lu 3
Lu 4
Lu 5
Lu 6
Lu 7
Lu 8
Lu 9
Lu 10
(Lu 11 Chin.)
Lu 7 Lu 9 Lu 10 (Lu 11 Chin.)
(Lu 11 Chin.)
Lu 11

Fig. 13

unilaterally on the *contralateral* side. The needle should not be inserted deeply, as otherwise the patient will feel dizzy. It is also a very important and frequently-used point.
Location: On the radial edge, just one fingerbreadth proximal to the head of the radius, that is, somewhat above the 3rd pulse palpation position.

Lu 9

Chinese name: **Taiyuan.** Lu 9 is the tonification point and source point at the same time. We use it primarily as a main point for all types of vascular disorders, arrhythmia, and states of agitation; less frequently for bronchitis and neuralgia in the thorax and arm. It is also used as a supplement is the treatment of enuresis nocturna.
Location: Lu 9 also lies on the radial edge on the level of the crease of the wrist, thus, somewhat distal to the 1st pulse palpation position.

Lu 11

Chinese name: **Shaoshang.** This point is "the Master Point of Disorders of the Throat." We use it symptomatically – for children perhaps only massaging with the fingernail – for all inflammations and pain in the pharynx and larynx, and also for bronchitis, sinusitis, and otitis. It is used less frequently for enteritis; often for writer's cramp. It is an important point for analgesia.
Location: Dorsal, 2 mm proximal and lateral to the corner of the cuticle of the thumb on the index finger side. Interestingly, recent Chinese articles describe this point as being on the medial side. However, the fact we were able to perform well over 100 tonsillectomies using Lu 11 in the *lateral location I have described,* together with LI 4, is more convincing than the Chinese reports. The Chinese performed their tonsillectomies using LI 4 and St 44 only.

THE MERIDIAN OF THE LARGE INTESTINE

The Meridian of the Large Intestine receives its energy from the Lung Meridian and passes it on to the Meridian of the Stomach. It is a YANG meridian. Abbreviations: English: LI, not to be confused with Li (Liver)! German: Di (Dickdarm); French: GI (Gros Intestin). Its pulse point is on the *right* wrist distal to the radial apophysis, however, this time in the *superficial* position. Its associated (concurring) point is B 25; its alarm point is St 25 on the midpoint of an imaginary line between the navel and the top of the iliac crest. The meridian begins 2 mm medial and proximal to the corner of the cuticle of the index finger (on the thumb side), travels dorsally upwards over the index finger and hand, gradually turning laterally on the forearm, and passes the elbow strictly laterally. It continues over the attachment of the deltoid to the acromion and from there over the lateral side of the neck to the nasolabial groove, ending on the upper end thereof (Fig. 14).

LI 1

Chinese name: **Shangjang.** LI 1 is the master point for toothache. It goes without saying that it is only used symptomatically. In particular, it is able to distinctly alleviate pain during a dental treatment. It is also used for acne therapy; less frequently for stomatitis, gingivitis. It is an important analgesia point.
Location: Dorsal, 2 mm proximal and medial to the corner of the cuticle of the index finger (on the thumb side).

LI 2

Chinese name: **Erjian.** This point is always used together with LI 3 (see below).
Location: On the skin crease which is formed when a fist is made enclosing the thumb, hence, just distal to the metacarpophalangeal joint of the index finger.

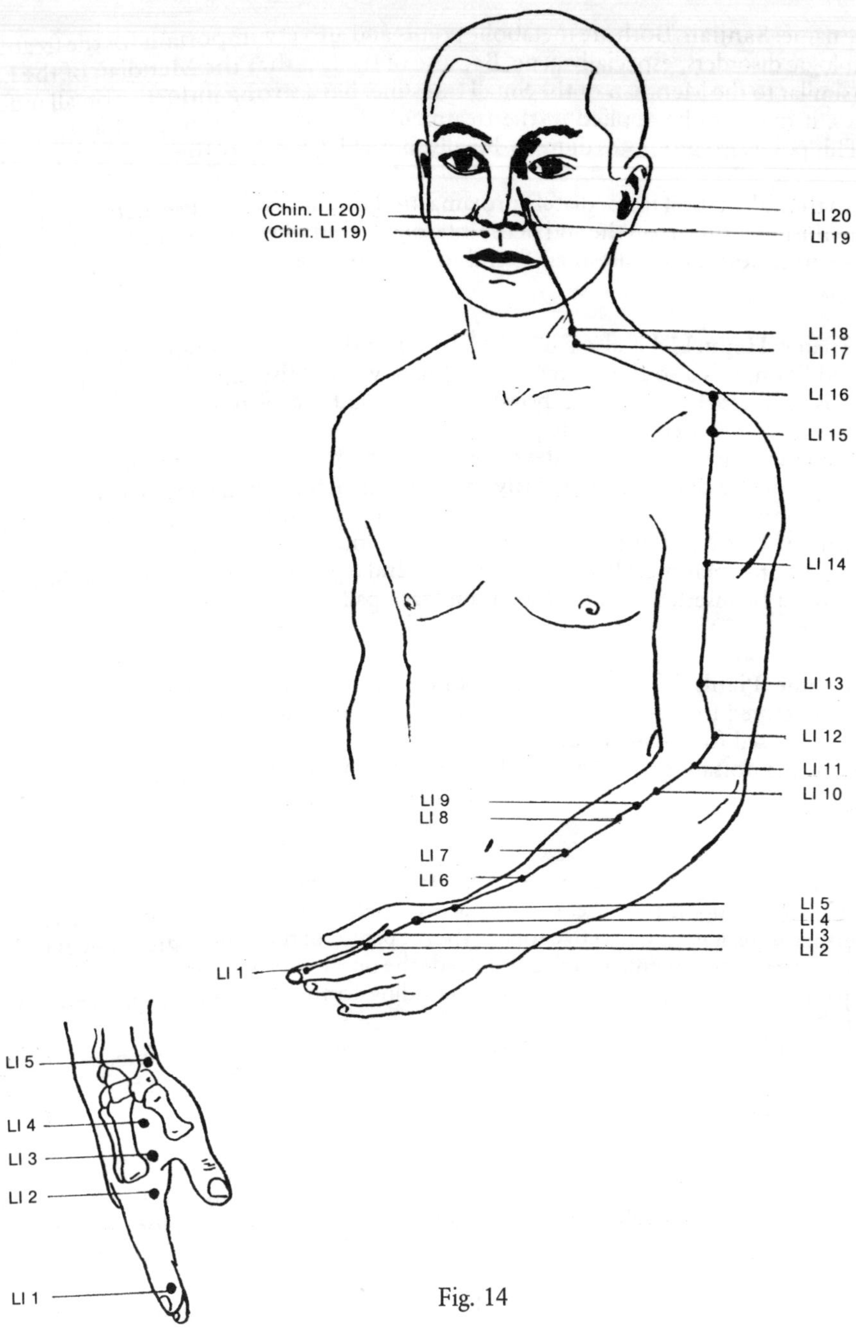
(Chin. LI 20)
(Chin. LI 19)
LI 20
LI 19
LI 18
LI 17
LI 16
LI 15
LI 14
LI 13
LI 12
LI 11
LI 10
LI 9
LI 8
LI 7
LI 6
LI 5
LI 4
LI 3
LI 2
LI 1
LI 5
LI 4
LI 3
LI 2
LI 1

Fig. 14

LI 3

Chinese name: **Sanjian.** Both are metabolic points and are very important for the treatment of dermatologic disorders, especially acne. Because of the fact that the Meridian of the Large Intestine (similar to the Meridian of the Small Intestine) has a strong influence on all mucous membranes, it may also be applied in the treatment of sinusitis, rhinitis, conjuctivitis, and enteritis. This point also promotes diuresis. Finally, both LI 2 and 3 are the meridian's sedation points.
Location: In the indentation immediately proximal to the joint cavity of the metacarpophalangeal joint of the index finger, on the end of the interdigital fold when the thumb is stretched out as far as possible. Both points are then found to be close to each other.

LI 4

Chinese name: **Hegu.** LI 4 is also a metabolic point and a very important therapeutic point at that. In addition, it is also the source point. Again, we find the same "mucous membrane disorders" as indicate LI 2 and 3, however, this point's action is even more intense. Furthermore, it is often used as remote point for the treatment of migraines and cephalaea. A common cold can be prevented from developing with this point. (The best time for treatment is during the prodromal stage, that is, shortly after the patient feels symptoms which, according to experience, mean that a cold will develop). If the cold has already become manifest, the effect is much slighter. This point also has a wide range of action in analgesia.
Location: In the proximal angle between the 1st and 2nd metacarpals on the back of the hand. The needle must be inserted towards the 2nd metacarpal!

LI 6

Chinese name: **Pianli.** LI 6 is the passage or Lo point to its partner organ, the Lung. It is mainly acupunctured for paresis of the upper extremity, especially of the thumb and index finger. It is also used for spastic intestinal disorders.
Location: On the dorsal, medial edge of the radius on the proximal end of the distal third thereof.

LI 10

Chinese name: **Shousanli.** (Sanli of the arm). It is also a test point for constipation if it is inadequately painful upon pressure. It is frequently used in the treatment of spastic constipation. Furthermore, it is very effective for all types of paresis of the upper extremities. It is also included in migraine treatment, as well as for headache on the crown of the head, and is often used for pain and paralysis in the areas corresponding to the trigeminal, facial, and radial nerves.
Location: LI 10 lies on the dorsal, lateral edge of the radius when the hand is supinated, on the distal end of the proximal third in the middle of the extensor musculature which begins there. It is easier to find than to describe because it is always sensitive to pressure.

LI 11

Chinese name: **Quichi.** LI 11 is the tonification point. It is especially effective for constipation, as well as for itching of the skin of unknown etiology. It is also used for paresis of the hands and arms; less frequently for hemiplegia. You will often find it worth your while to use this point for furunculosis and eczema.
Location: When the arm is maximally bent, LI 11 lies on the lateral end of the crease of the elbow.

LI 12

Chinese name: **Zhouliao.** For brachial neuralgia and difficulty in lifting the arm to the side, together with

LI 13
Chinese name: **Wuli.** Same indications as LI 12; they are used together.
Location: On thc proximal ends of the lower and middle thirds respectively of the distance between LI 11 and LI 14.

LI 14
Chinese name: **Binao.** This point is used for pain in the shoulder and as adjuvant in the treatment of all types of pain and paresis of the upper extremities.
Location: On the lowest point of attachment of the deltoid muscle on the upper arm.

LI 15
Chinese name: **Jianyu.** LI 15 is the master point for all types of paresis of the upper extremity and also for all types of neuralgia and rheumatic complaints in this area and in the shoulder girdle. It is used less frequently for hypertension.
Location: On the lateral edge of the shoulder in the indentation below the acromion.

LI 16
Chinese name: **Jugu.** LI 16 lies on the tip – of the acromion. It is used as a supplement in the treatment of paralyses, shoulder pain, and arthritis.

LI 19
Chinese name: **Heliao.** LI 19, together with LI 20, is the main point for treatment of the nose. We use it to the same extent in the treatment of colds, sinusitis, vasomotor rhinitis, and anosmia. However, it is also used occasionally for constipation and headache. Also, it is rarely omitted in the treatment of trigeminal neuralgia.
Location: In the nasolabial groove on the level of the nostrils.

LI 20
Chinese name: **Yingyiang.** Same indications, same usage.
Location: On the upper end of the nasolabial groove, or rather, in the angle of the os nasale and maxilla. These points are quite painful and should always be acupunctured first.

Chinese reports indicate that LI 19 and 20 cross over to the opposite side. Because of the fact that these points are usually acupunctured bilaterally anyway, this point of view does not seem to me to be relevant; likewise, the slightly different location does not appear to be of importance.

THE MERIDIAN OF THE STOMACH

The Meridian of the Stomach receives its energy from the Meridian of the Large Intestine and passes it on to the Meridian of the Spleen-Pancreas. It is a YANG meridian. Abbreviations: English: St; German: M (Magen); French: E (Estomac). Its pulse point is over the radial apophysis of the *right* wrist in the *superficial* position. Its associated (concurring) point is B 21; its alarm point is CV 12 (a good 2 fingerbreadths distal to the tip of the xiphoid on the ventral midline). The meridian begins on the upper edge of the temporal fossa, travels distally to the mandible, extends upwards to below the eye, travels distally again to the middle of the clavicula and then downwards along the mammillary line, approching the Kidney Meridian in the region of the abdomen, then travels ventrally along the thigh over the knee and then more laterally over the leg, arriving at its end point via the dorsum pedis. Its end point is 2 mm lateral and proximal to the lateral corner of the cuticle of the 2nd toe (Fig. 15).

The beginning points up to St 8 are numbered differently in newer Chinese data.

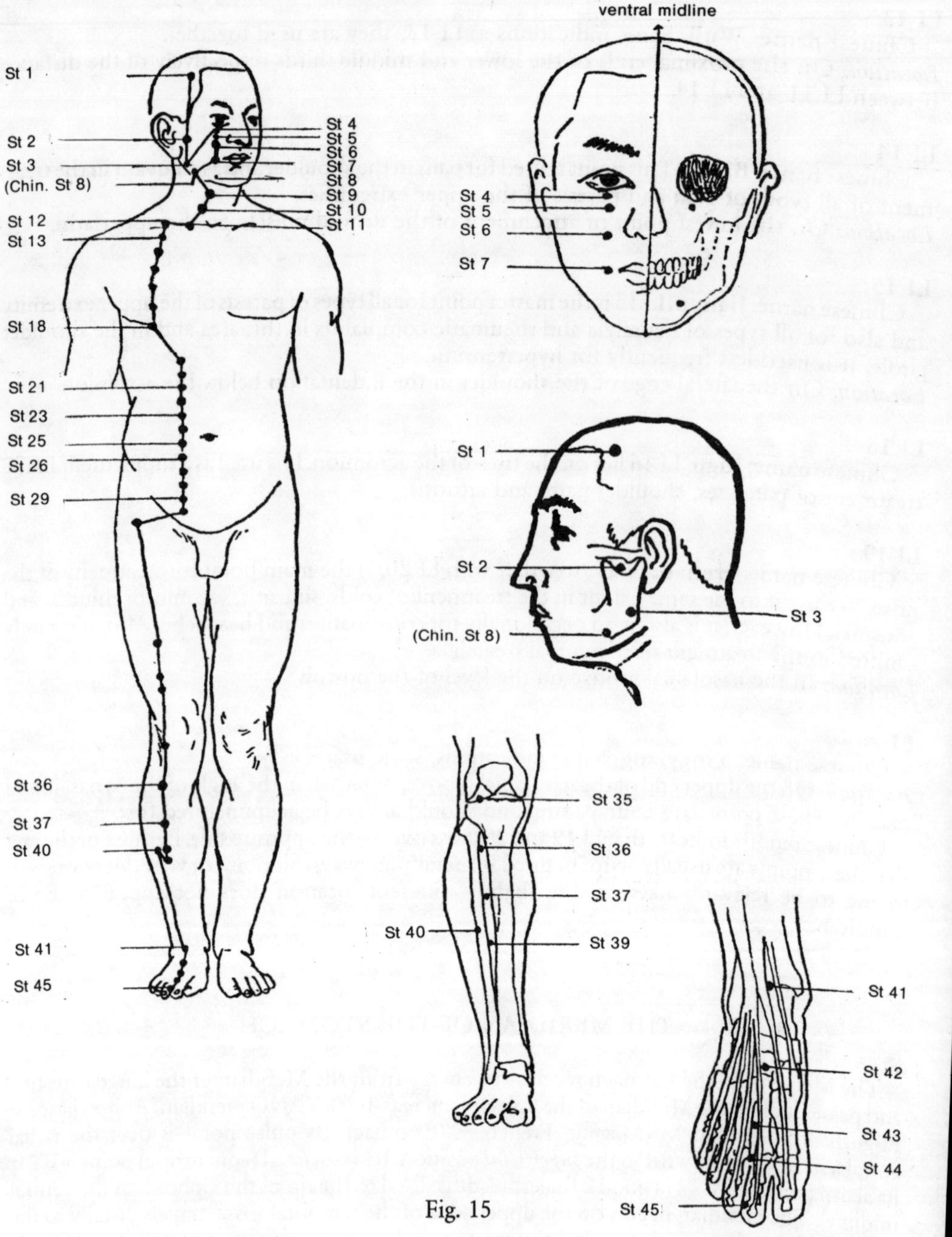
ventral midline
St 1
St 2
St 3
(Chin. St 8)
St 4
St 5
St 6
St 7
St 8
St 9
St 10
St 11
St 12
St 13
St 18
St 21
St 23
St 25
St 26
St 29
St 35
St 36
St 37
St 39
St 40
St 41
St 42
St 43
St 44
St 45

Fig. 15

St 1

Chinese name: **Touwei.** St 1 is used as supplement in the treatment of headache and sometimes for trigeminal neuralgia of the first branch.
Location: On the upper edge of the temporal fossa, about 4 fingerbreadths above and one fingerbreadth behind the angle of the orbit of the eye and cheek bone.

St 2

Chinese name: **Xiaguan.** This point is frequently used for facial paralysis, trigeminal neuralgia, and tics; occasionally for headache and sinusitis.
Location: In the middle of the attachment of the masseter on the cheek bone.

St 3

Chinese name: **Jiache.** This point is used for the above indications and also for stuttering and peroral cutaneous efflorescence.
Location: On the attachment of the masseter on the upper edge of the mandible, usually on the angle of the jaw; less frequently (usually in prognathism) in front of it.

St 4

Chinese name: **Chengqi.** St 4 is used very rarely for facial paralysis and trigeminal neuralgia. It lies on the lower edge of the orbit of the eye on an imaginary perpendicular line through the middle of the pupil. Acupuncture of this point requires a very steady hand. Caution!

St 6

Chinese name: **Juliao.** St 6 and its neighboring points, 7 and 8, have the same indications, that is, sinusitis, stuttering, tics, facial paralysis, and trigeminal neuralgia. They can be acupunctured together or individually.
Location: They all lie on an imaginary perpendicular line through the middle of the pupil. St 6 lies on the point of intersection with the nostril. Farther distal you will find

St 7

Chinese name: **Dicang** on the point of intersection with the corner of the mouth and

St 8

Chinese name: **Daying** on the point of intersection with the lower edge of the mandible.

St 10

Chinese name: **Shiutu.** St 10 is an important point for the treatment of vocal fatigue and hoarseness in speakers and singers, however, it also has considerable influence on the thyroid. Furthermore, it alleviates stomach spasms.
Location: On the frontal edge of the sternocleidomastoid muscle on the level of the thyroid cartilage, lateral to the center thereof.

St 12

Chinese name: **Quepen.** St 12 is an important stomach point (*Virchow's* node). We use it for all stomach symptoms such as belching, heartburn, nausea, and spasm, as well as for intolerance of wine.
Location: On the upper edge of the clavicula between the points of attachment of the sternocleidomastoid.

St 13

Chinese name: **Qihu.** St 13 is also called the second locus of St 12, however, on the lower edge of the clavicle.

St 18

This point is simultaneously the point Li 14 and has already been discussed in that section.

St 21

Chinese name: **Liangmen.** St 21 is frequently used in the treatment of spastic colitis, all types of digestive disorders, gastric and duodenal ulcers, and often for neurodystonia.
Location: In the angle of the 8th intercostal space; may often be found 1 fingerbreadth medial thereto.

St 23

Chinese name: **Taiyi.** An important point for the treatment of gastric and duodenal ulcers.
Location: On the chondro-osseous junction of the 9th rib; often 1 fingerbreadth medial thereto.

St 25

Chinese name: **Tianshu.** St 25 is the alarm point of the Large Intestine. We use it for constipation, tympanism, and nausea; less frequently for heartburn and stomach pains. It is also used in acupuncture analgesia.
Location: Midway between the navel and the anterior superior iliac crest; in Chinese data, 2 fingerbreadths lateral to the navel, possibly because of the different pelvic structure and length of the intestine of Asiatics.

St 26

Chinese name: **Wailing.** Used for all types of abdominal spasm.
Location: Approximately midway between the navel and the anterior superior iliac spine.

St 29

Chinese name: **Guilai.** St 29 is mainly used for constipation, tympanism, less frequently for ulcers. It is also used for adnexia and dysmenorrhea.
Location: 2 fingerbreadths above the upper edge of the pubic bone, 2 fingerbreadths lateral to the symphysis *(McBurney's* point).

St 30

Chinese name: **Qichong.** St 30 is used for dyspepsia, tympanism, and anorexia, as well as for adnexitis, frigidity, and impotence. It also serves to facilitate childbirth and is used in the treatment of women with back pain which worsens at night.
Location: This point is found 2 fingerbreadths lateral to the symphysis on the upper edge of the pubic bone, and the needle is inserted downwards.

St 31

Chinese name: **Biguan.** Identical to Li 12 which has already been dealt with.

St 36

Chinese name: **Zusanli** (compare LI 10: "Sanli" of the arm, Zusanli: "Sanli" of the leg.) This is a very important acupuncture point. Its epithet is "Godly Equanimity." Hence, its psychological indications which are very appropriately described by the concept of "Asiatic serenity". It is effective for irritability as well as for melancholia; for stagefright and shyness, as well as for delusions of grandeur. Furthermore, it has a wide range of action on the genital organs and hormonal equilibrium, as well as on all changes in blood pressure. It is also used effectively for skin diseases. Its literal meaning is "three villages". Therefore, it was, and is, used to increase the capacity for walking (marching), as well as for therapy of all types of spasms, paralysis, or pain in the lower extremities. Of course, it also has a broad spectrum of action for

all abdominal disorders or illnesses and, in connection therewith, for headaches and migraines. It is one of the points with the widest scope of action, and is rarely omitted from a treatment. It is also called "the great healer of the knees and feet"; it is particularly effective for swelling in those areas. An important point for analgesia!
Location: On the point of intersection of lines half a fingerbreadth lateral to the linea interossea of the tibia and 2 fingerbreadths below the head of the fibula, thus, between the m. tibialis anterior and m. extensor digit. longus.

Appendix Point (St 36-01)
This point does not lie exactly on the Meridian of the Stomach, and corresponds more closely to the Chinese point "Lanwei", however, I consider it deserving of mention. Being a surgeon myself, it goes against my grain to say that in an emergency, acupuncturing this point alleviates acute appendicitis, although it is often done effectively in China. In certain cases, we can consider it feasible, however, I see the point's main significance in regard to diagnosis, especially in children who dissimulate, or persons who are hyposensitive or insensitive to pain, which is not at all rare. If this point is distinctly painful, I consider its implications more important than some less clear, conventional findings.
Location: This point lies on the m. tibialis anterior, about 2½ fingerbreadths below the angle between the tibia and the fibula, and is usually more painful on the right than on the left, though it can be clearly identified on both sides. Roughly sketched, it is located about 2 fingerbreadths below St 36.

St 40
Chinese name: **Fenglong.** St 40 is the passage or Lo point to the partner meridian, the Meridian of the Spleen-Pancreas. It is used for abdominal complaints, especially spasm, particularly when the body is cool and moist. Furthermore, it is used for singultus (hiccoughs) and non-localized pain in the stomach and chest.
Location: On the frontal edge of the fibula, 1 fingerbreadth above the midpoint between the anterior tibial tubercle and the lateral malleolus.

St 41
Chinese name: **Jiexi.** St 41 is the tonification point. We use it for atonic constipation, and hyposecretion of the stomach with tympanism; locally, for arthritis in the foot and ankle, less frequently for acne.
Location: On the lower edge of the tibia in the middle of the tarsus.

St 42
Chinese name: **Chongyang.** St 42 is the source point. It is used for hyper as well as hypoacidity of the stomach, for constipation and tympanism; less frequently for spasm. It is also effective for paralysis of the leg and as an adjuvant in the treatment of facial paralysis. It has a calming influence on the psyche.
Location: Somewhat distal to St 41 over the joint of the navicular bone with the 2nd and 3rd cuneiform bones.

St 44
Chinese name: **Neiting.** Main point for treatment of nightmares and enuresis nocturna, as well as an important analgesia point.
Location: Proximal, in the angle of the metatarsophalangeal joints of the 2nd and 3rd toes.

St 45
Chinese name: **Lidui**; literally, "the gruesome payment", which gives an indication of how painful acupuncture of this point can be. It is mainly used for hyperacidity and hypersecretion

of the stomach, however, also for alternating diarrhea and constipation. It often has a favorable remote action on rhinitis and headache. Sedation point.
Location: 2 mm proximal and lateral to the corner of the cuticle of the 2nd toe, dorsal.

THE MERIDIAN OF THE SPLEEN-PANCREAS

The Meridian of the Spleen-Pancreas receives its energy from the Meridian of the Stomach and passes it on to the Meridian of the Heart. It is a YIN meridian. Abbreviations: English: SP; German: MP (Milz-Pankreas); French: RP (Rate-Pancreas). Its associated (concurring) point is B 20. Its pulse point is on the *right* wrist over the radial apophysis, however, this time in the *deep* position. The meridian begins 2 mm medial and proximal to the outside corner of the cuticle of the big toe, travels along the inner side of the instep to the posterior edge of the tibia, passes the knee strictly medially, and follows the sartorius muscle along the thigh. It ascends over the abdomen as the most lateral ventral meridian up to the 2nd intercostal space, 2 fingerbreadths lateral to the mammilla, and drops from there to its end point in the 6th intercostal space on the frontal axillary line. Therewith, the third cycle of energy is closed and the circulation of energy begins again with the Meridian of the Heart. Here, again, the alternation centrifugal-centripetal, centrifugal-centripetal, or the course: lateral chest wall – fingers; fingers – head; head – toes; and toes – lateral wall of the chest (Fig. 16).

SP 2

Chinese name: **Dadu.** SP 2 is the tonification point. Its main indication is drowsiness during the day and cold hands and feet; abdomimal spasms and exhaustion as well.
Location: On the medial side of the articulation of the metatarsophalangeal joint of the big toe.

SP 3

Chinese name: **Taibai.** SP 3 is the source point. We use it for abdominal spasms as well as neuralgia and paresis of the lower extremities. It is also very effective for general weakness.
Location: On the tendon of the hallucal abductor on the inner edge of the foot just proximal to the metatarsophalangeal joint of the big toe.

SP 4

Chinese name: **Gongsun.** Another cardinal point which is simultaneously the meridian's passage point to its partner organ, the Stomach. It is our main point for diarrhea, spasm in the lower abdomen, and tympanism. It is also helpful in combatting fatigue, for angina pectoris, and facilitates childbirth. It is frequently used.
Location: On the inner edge of the joint between the 1st metatarsal and 1st cuneiform bones, somewhat proximal thereto.

SP 5

Chinese name: **Shangqui.** SP 5 is the sedation point and also the master point for all types of "connective tissue weakness" (for which the meridian is particularly responsible). It is also important for all types of circulatory disorders. We use this point especially to achieve immediate alleviation of pain from varicose veins. Of course, acupuncture cannot in any way change the varicose veins themselves. Furthermore, usually together with Lu 7, this point eliminates swelling such as that caused by the varicose symptom complex, or after thrombophlebitis. It is also helpful for treatment of the so-called cellulitis. As far as connective tissue weakness is concerned, it is not only used for disorders such as varicose veins, hemorrhoids, all types of prolapse and ptosis, but also for distended patients and those who always feel chilly or cold, sleepy during the day, dejected, and have a defeatist attitude. Of

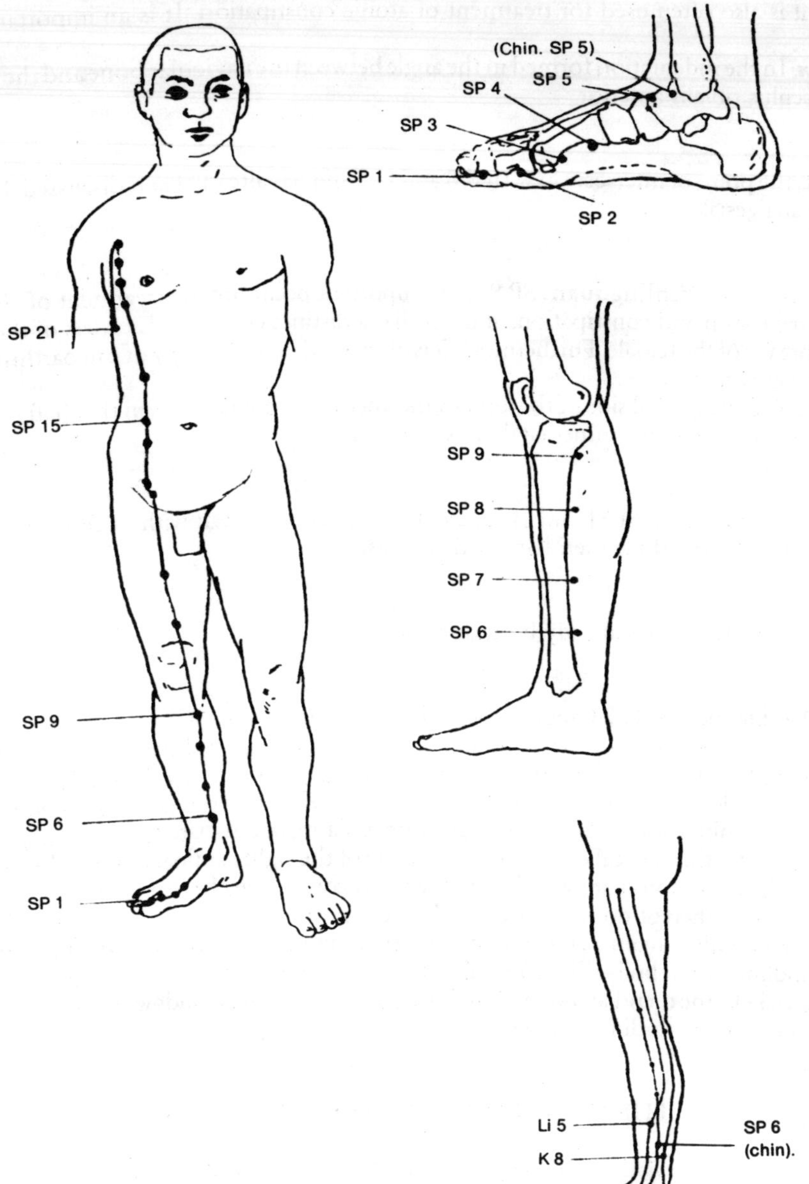
(Chin. SP 5)
SP 5
SP 4
SP 3
SP 1
SP 2
SP 21
SP 15
SP 9
SP 6
SP 1
SP 9
SP 8
SP 7
SP 6
Li 5
K 8
SP 6
(chin).

Fig. 16

course, it is also often used for treatment of atonic constipation. It is an important, general point.
Location: In the indentation formed in the angle between the navicular bone and the tendon of the musculus tibialis anterior.

SP 6

SP 6 is the point of intersection with K 8 and Li 5 and has already been discussed. Important also for analgesia!

SP 9

Chinese name: **Yinlingquan.** SP 9 is an important point for the treatment of all types of abdominal spasm and constipation, and also has a distinct effect on disorders of the internal genital organs of the female. Furthermore, it is often used in the therapy of osteoarthritits of the knee and gonarthritis.
Location: On the medial side of the joint of the knee in the angle between the shaft of the tibia and the medial condyle, immediately next to Li 9.

SP 11a

SP 11a is identical to St 31 and Li 12, and has already been dealt with. It coincides with the zone formed by the three meridians at this locus.

SP 15

Identical to Li 13; has already been discussed.

SP 21

SP 21 is identical to G 24 and has been listed in that section.

We have now concluded the third and last cycle of energy and have arrived back at the Meridian of the Heart. We have discussed all 12 partner, bilateral meridans or "Kings". There are also 8 so-called "wonder meridians", which travel over parts of one or several meridians, and do not have tonification, sedation, passage, source, alarm, or associated (concurring) points of their own, but rather, are called into action via one of the eight cardinal points. They are more suitably called "extraordinary vessels" or "Mos". Of course, they have no pulse points of their own. Only two thereof do not correspond to any portions of meridians with which we are familiar, and both contain a large number of very important points. They are the ventral and dorsal midlines of the body. Therefore, all of the points of these two vessels described below are not bilateral like the meridian points, but rather, each point corresponds with one and only one locus. The first extraordinary vessel is

THE CONCEPTION VESSEL OR JENN-MO

We use the abbreviation CV. The German abbreviation is KG (Konzeptionsgefäß); the French is VC (Vaisseau Conception). This is the ventral midline; the vessel begins at the anus and ascends over the symphysis and navel to the xiphoid and on over the sternum and the incisura jugularis, passes the thyroid cartilage and ends above the chin. We believe that the energy ascends in this vessel, and therefore begin at the bottom (Fig. 17).

CV 1

Chinese name: **Huiyin.** CV 1 is a very effective point for all sexual indications and genital disorders. The Chinese also warm the needle before inserting it into this point. However, because of its somewhat problematic location, it is used less frequently than it deserves to be.
Location: Immediately in front of and above the anus.

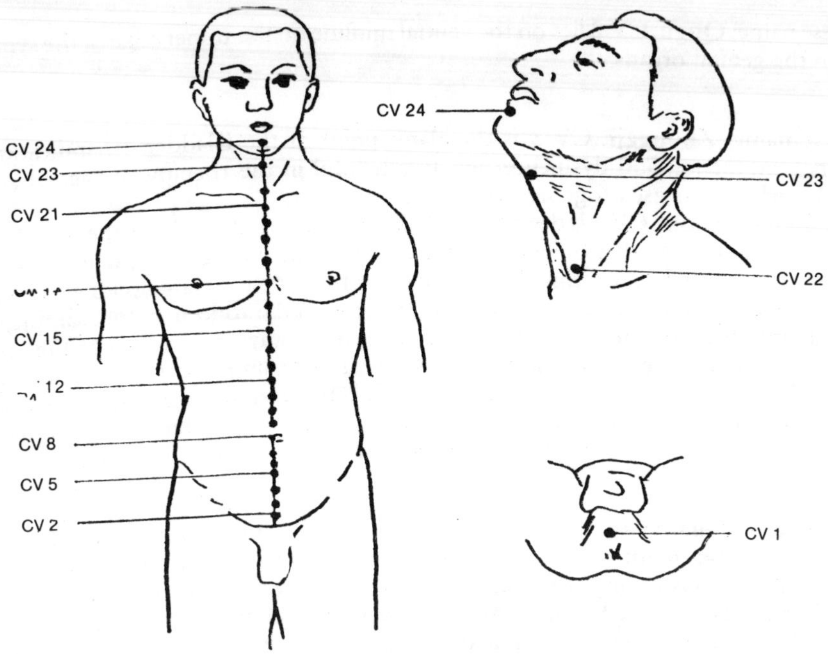

Fig. 17

CV 2

Chinese name: **Qugu.** CV 2 lies on the ventral midline on the upper edge of the symphysis. It acts on the genital organs.

CV 3

Chinese name: **Zhonggji.** CV 3 is the alarm point of the Bladder. Its indications are: pollakiuria, impotence, and dysmenorrhea. It is helpful in the therapy of vaginal and anal pruritus for which it is used together with CV 1 and PV 1.
Location: In most books, CV 3 is described as being 2 fingerbreadths above the symphysis (on the midline of course, like all subsequent points). That is absolutely correct, at least in regard to this point. However, when locating the next point at the lastest, we are no longer able to use exclusively this unit of measurement, as indeed, the form of the abdomen, for example, a beer-belly, or a sagging abdomen in elderly persons, does not always correspond to the idealized lines on charts. Therefore, my friend and co-worker, *Feucht,* and I suggest another method, which I wish to use here in the assumption that it is better and more practical. To locate the points CV 3-7, we divide the distance between the symphysis and the navel into five parts. Thus, our CV 3 lies on the proximal end of the first fifth above the symphysis.

CV 4

Chinese name: **Guanyuan.** CV 4 is the alarm point of the Small Intestine. We use it for all intestinal spasms and enteritis, especially when accompanied by marked, general weakness. All gynecological disorders having symptoms of weakness are treated via this point. Finally, it is also used for headaches which worsen during movement and improve at rest.
Location: The position is the same as that of CV 3, however, two-fifths above the symphysis.

CV 5

Chinese name: **Shimen.** CV 5 is the main alarm point of the Triple Heater. It influences all three of the functions which that meridian represents, and is hence used for menstrual disorders, dyspepsia, and asthma.
Location: Three-fifths above the symphysis.

CV 6

Chinese name: **Qihai,** the "Sea of Energy". CV 6 is one of the most important acupuncture points. It is very effective in the treatment of all states of exhaustion or insufficiency. One of its indications whets the beginner's appetite for learning acupuncture: vertigo upon looking upwards. As soon as the needle has been inserted into this point, the patient can look upwards as long as he likes without difficulty and maintains this ability even after the needle has been removed. This is a common complaint, especially among housewives, therefore, it is worth-while making this one of your first practical acupuncture experiences. This point is also effective for constipation, tympanism, chills, and insomnia. It is also called "the Sea of Fertility", a fact of which you should make younger patients aware should the point be used for a purpose unrelated to this epithet. Furthermore, it is an important point for all other types of vertigo including *Menière's* disease. Catatonic patients are frequently given a pre-treatment with this point, several metabolic points, and possibly some other fortifying points before actual therapy is begun.
Location: CV 6 lies in the middle of the fourth fifth above the symphysis; on thin persons, 2 fingerbreadths below the navel.

CV 7

Chinese name: **Yinjiao.** CV 7 is the lower (sexual) alarm point of the Triple Heater. It is used for all types of sexual hyperfunction and adnexitis.
Location: On the proximal end of the fourth fifth above the symphysis, or 1 fingerbreadth below the navel.

CV 9

Chinese name: **Shuifen.** CV 9 is an important point for treatment of all purulent inflammations, especially furuncles; occasionally for spastic constipation as well.
Location: Here, too, we recommend dividing the distance between the navel and the tip of the xiphoid into 8 parts. CV 9 thus lies one-eighth above the navel. On thin persons, this corresponds to one fingerbreadth.

CV 12

Chinese name: **Zhongwan.** CV 12 is the alarm point of the Stomach and also the middle (digestive) alarm point of the Triple Heater. It is used in the therapy of meteorism and tympanism, particularly in the upper abdomen, as well as for dyspepsia and ulcers.
Location: Exactly midway between the navel and the xiphoid.

CV 13

Chinese name: **Shangwan.** CV 13 is a special point for all types of spastic stomach disorders. We use it for ulcers and gastritis, as well as for all types of colic and anorexia. It is often included in the treatment of *Roemheld's* syndrome and angina pectoris.
Location: Three-eighths below the tip of the xiphoid.

CV 14

Chinese name: **Jujue.** CV 14 is the alarm point of the Heart. It is used for all types of precardiac pain, tachycardia, and angina pectoris, and especially for hyperemesis gravidarum.
Location: One-eighth below the xiphoid.

CV 15

Chinese name: **Juwei.** Another very important point. *Bachmann* describes it along with PV 19 as "the Bellergal® of acupuncture". It has an excellent effect on all types of psychasthenia, the so-called manager's syndrome, and all states of exhaustion caused by mental tension. It is also frequently included in treatment of all migraine cases. Furthermore, we add it to the point programs for ulcers, colitis, and all types of spastic processes in the digestive tract. Finally, it is very valuable in the treatment of impotence and ejaculatio praecox.
Location: Just below the tip of the xiphoid.

CV 17

Chinese name: **Shanzhong.** Yet another very important point. It is the upper, or respiratory, alarm point of the Triple Heater. It is effective for all types of disorders in the thorax, especially bronchial asthma, Roemheld's syndrome, precardiac pain and all types of sensations of constriction in the heart region. It is also frequently used for intercostal neuralgia.
Location: In the middle of the sternum on the level of the 4th intercostal space.

CV 21

Chinese name: **Xuanji.** CV 21 is our main point for heartburn and (nervous) tickling cough; less frequently for bronchitis.
Location: In the incisura jugularis on the posterior (inner) edge of the sternum.

CV 22

Tiantu is its Chinese name. It is effective for heartburn and hoarseness, however, its regulative action on the thyroid is particularly noteworthy.

THE PILOT (OR GOVERNOR) VESSEL OR TOU-MO

The Pilot Vessel follows the dorsal midline of the body. Like the Conception Vessel, it starts at the anus, however, behind and above it, travels upwards over the tips of the spinous processes of all vertebrae, traverses the head and nose in the midline and ends on the philtrum of the upper lip. In this vessel as well, the energy ascends; the two currents of energy from JENN-MO and TOU-MO meet perorally via secondary vessels. Like JENN-MO, this vessel has no tonification etc. points of its own. We use the abbreviation PV (Pilot Vessel) or GV (Governor Vessel). In German the abbreviation is LG (Lenkergefäß) or GG (Gouverneurgefäß); in French it is VG (Vaisseau Gouverneur). Newer Chinese data diverge considerably regarding this vessel. This is due to the fact that the Chinese usually insert the needle much deeper into these points than we do with the intention of nearing the dura. Therefore, they insert the needle below the spinous process, which accounts for the discrepancies in levels of the points' locations. We do not recommend using such needling methods for forensic reasons.

PV 1

Chinese name: **Changqiang.** As mentioned in regard to CV 1, this point can be acupunctured with a heated needle; it is also a sexual point and is effective for anal pruritus and anal eczema. However, it is rarely used because of its.
Location: Just behind the anal orifice.

PV 2

Chinese name: **Yaoshu.** PV 2 is on the dorsal midline between the coccyx and sacrum. It is effective for lumbago, sciatica, as well as for menstrual disorders and expediates childbirth.

PV 3

Chinese name: **Yaoyangguan.** Used for all types of neuralgia and pain following trauma, also for cerebral concussion.
Location: On the tip of the spinous process (like all following points) of L 5.

PV 4

Chinese name: **Mingmen.** PV 4 is the most important sexual point in acupuncture. Furthermore, it is frequently used for lumbago and general exhaustion; less frequently for anemia. If this point is acupunctured for lumbago, you should make the patient aware of possible changes (both negative and positive) in regard to sex.
Location: PV 4 lies on L 3, hence, relatively deep if the spinous process is closely observed.

PV 6

Chinese name: **Jizhong.** PV 6 lies on the spinous process of L 1. Its neighbor (6a) lies on the 12th thoracic vertebra. Both are acupunctured for restlessness and general weakness, as well as for developmental disturbances in children.

PV 9

Chinese name: **Lingtai.** PV 9 is the point for mental and physical weakness in children and is used for all types of developmental disturbances.
Location: On the 8th thoracic vertebra.

PV 10

Chinese name: **Shendao.** PV 10 lies on the 6th thoracic vertebra; the point 10a on the 5th thoracic vertebra, always on the tip of the spinous process. Both are used for psychasthenia, developmental disorders in children; less frequently for local spondylarthritic pain.

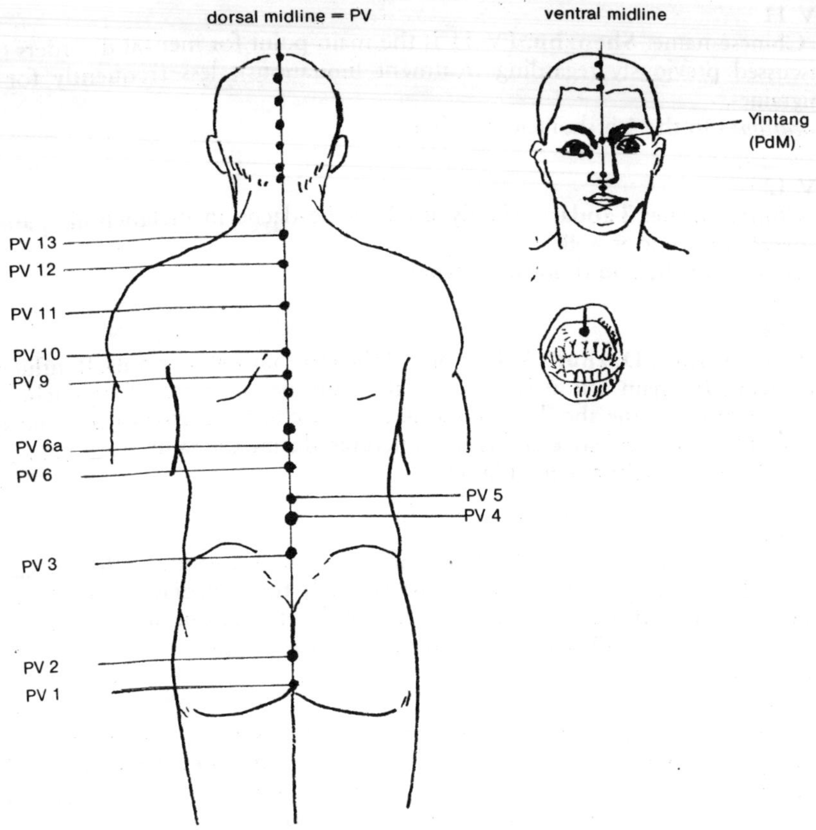
dorsal midline = PV
ventral midline
Yintang
(PdM)
PV 13
PV 12
PV 11
PV 10
PV 9
PV 6a
PV 6
PV 5
PV 4
PV 3
PV 2
PV 1

Fig. 18

PV 11

Chinese name: **Shenzhu.** PV 11 is the main point for mental disorders (which we have discussed previously regarding treatment limitations); less frequently for headache and migraines.
Location: On the 4th thoracic vertebra.

PV 12

Chinese name: **Taodao.** Mainly used for headache in melancholic patients; often for cervical syndrome as well.
Location: On the 2nd thoracic vertebra.

PV 13

Chinese name: **Dazhui.** PV 13 is one of the most important ponts. It influences all YANG meridians. Its main action is on cervical syndrome, all types of headache, neuralgia and inflammations in the shoulder and arm, and for complete exhaustion. The supplementary point, 13a, is also effective and is acupunctured during the same treatment. Reunion point!
Location: On C 7; the point 13a on C 6.

PV 16

Chinese name: **Fengfu.** PV 16 is our main point for regulation of the pituitary gland. It has an excellent effect on all menstrual disorders and dysfunction of the thyroid and other internal secretory glands. It is also useful in the treatment of headache and migraines.
Location: On the midline, on the lower edge of the occiput.

PV 19

Chinese name: **Houding.** As already said, together with CV 15, this very important point has an effect similar to Bellergal®. Furthermore, it increases the ability to concentrate, is effective for insomnia, migraines, and headache, as well as for sinusitis, rhinitis, and vertigo.
Location: On the midline on the point of intersection of the lambdoid and sagittal sutures in the indentation. Warning: Do not insert the needle too far!

PV 20

Chinese name: **Baihui (Pae Roe).** PV 20 is effective for headache, sinusitis, and ophthalmic disorders. According to Chinese literature, it is equivalent to PV 19, which is correct.
Location: On the midline on the highest point of the crown.

PV 23

Chinese name: **Shenting.** Acts on the mucous membrane and is also effective for vertigo.
Location: On the midline on the forehead at the hairline, or where it once was.

Point de Merveille (also called Yintang):

The Point de Merveille is sometimes referred to as PV 25. It is an important point for sinusitis and headache, and is also used for anosmia. It immediately enables free breathing through the nose. It is also often used together with B 2 as the frontal "magic" triangle for the same indications. An important point! It is the most important point in the frontal region of the skull, generally speaking as well.
Location: In the middle of the root of the nose.

PV 27

Chinese name: **Yinjiao.** Used for gingivitis.
Location: On the midline through the gums of the maxilla.

Thus, we see that the Pilot Vessel has predominately somatic indications in its lower portion only; above the 8th thoracic vertebra, it corresponds to the psyche, and we only find somatic indications again on the head.

That concludes the discussion of the points which are important for a medical practice. I have limited myself to brief information mainly in order to give you a general view of the material. I have purposely left out all other points which are not needed as often. They are discussed in detail in more comprehensive works. Discussion of problems and individual results is also encouraged by the various acupuncture societies in courses and meetings, as well as at national and international congresses.

The individual reader will soon become more interested in acupuncture, in pulse diagnosis, and will continue to study. However, this little book will always serve as a foundation; having acquired this knowledge, he can begin practicing acupuncture, especially if he observes the following rules:

1. Start with simpler cases.

2. Do not insert too many needles during one treatment.

3. Discontinue treatment at the right time.

4. Always take influential factors into consideration, especially when they are discovered spontaneously or mentioned by the patient.

5. Always try to use pulse diagnosis, even for seemingly clear indications.

6. Always consult an appropriate specialist for complicated cases and have all necessary tests made.

7. Do not acupuncture the points I have singled out if the patient is menstruating or pregnant. Never acupuncture a patient too soon after x-ray or radium therapy or after spa treatment.

8. Do not become careless if your treatments are more successful than those of your colleagues who do not practice acupuncture.

I have always tried to express myself simply, have repeated some things in order to avoid confusion, and to make acupuncture easily comprehensible. The results you will achieve with acupuncture make the effort of learning it worthwhile.

Chapter VIII

RESEARCH ON ACUPUNCTURE

Is acupuncture really a useful method, and is it worthwhile for a modern physician trained in natural science to learn it? The question can only be answered with a loud and clear "yes", not lastly in view of the countless publications on the subject, which have already appeared all over the world in medical and scientific journals of high international repute. Nevertheless, there are still some confirmed adversaries to the method, such as *Dotzauer* and *Prokop,* in whose eyes acupuncture still belongs in the realm of occultism, mesmerism, and hypnosis, regardless of there being sufficient evidence disproving their theory.

In this section, I would like to summarize the significant results of research on acupuncture, which have been internationally acknowledged and published in medical and scientific journals. It comes as no surprise that the majority thereof deal with pain (that is, acupuncture analgesia), it being the most spectacular aspect.

Research on Acupuncture Analgesia

Especially after acupuncture analgesia had been ventured in the Occident (we used acupuncture analgesia for tonsillectomies, no other medication having been administered, with the exception of the usual preparatory measures prior to surgery, in early March, 1972), research mainly focused on neurophysiology. New light was shed on hitherto recognized pain-inhibiting phenomena, such as those achieved by vibration *(Keidel)* or various conduction velocities of the A-δ and C-fibers *(Foerster, Zottermann).* Likewise, agreement was soon reached in regard to the switching locations and putative areas in which acupuncture analgesia is effective. The first to be investigated was the respective corresponding section of the dorsal horn in the substantia gelatinosa Rolandi (hence, the switching location from the first to the second neuron); the second, in the thalamic nuclei. In animal experiments, *Chiang* was able to demonstrate the particular significance of the nucleus parafascicularis.

In collaboration with *Baum, Benzer, Pauser, Reichman,* and *Thoma,* we carried out numerous investigations in order to study the analgesic effect of acupuncture. To this end, an instrument was designed to introduce a needle into the skin of test persons at a constant velocity. If the proband perceived the pain as intolerable, he could remove the needle, it being fastened to the piston of a record syringe, at once via vacuum. The level reached was recorded on an arbitrary scale ranging from 0-2,500.

Every proband underwent three different tests: 1. without any analgesia whatsoever, 2. with acupuncture analgesia, 3. with pseudo-acupuncture, that is, intentional acupuncture of inappropriate skin loci. The experiment was a double-blind study. After the test, a group of psychologists carried out an investigation on these test persons using the Minnesota rating score. The result was astonishing: In contrast to the first test, the second and third tests revealed a distinct rise of the pain threshold. There was a difference between tests 2 and 3, it, however, being insignificant. It was the psychological test that significantly established the probands' perception of pain during tests 2 and 3 in favor of correctly applied acupuncture analgesia.

Kothbauer did a similar experiment on cows, making incisions and subsequently, sutures on the udder teats. In contrast to man, the untreated animal responded identically to the animal treated with pseudo-acupuncture – with massive defensive reactions, rendering the planned intervention impossible. In contrast thereto, the entire operation could be performed on several animals, these responding with no defensive reactions, when true acupuncture, and no other medication, was applied. The only reaction observed was that the whole udder was pulled up reflexly when touched in any way. Acupuncture analgesia in humans had already revealed that reflexes cannot be influenced via acupunctue. In collaboration, *Zimmermann* et al. and *Pauser* et al. demonstrated measurable discharges of nociceptive potentials of dorsal horn units in the spinal cord upon application of peripheral, standardized nociceptive stimuli to a receptor field on the pad of the hind limb of anesthetized cats with heat up to 50°C. These discharges greatly increased after three seconds, and only slowly diminished even after the ten-second stimulation, only to massively increase again spontaneously twelve seconds after the end of stimulation as an expression of after-sensation.

The same experiment, using, however, electric stimulation of the appropriately acupunctured point, revealed a significant reduction of discharges of nociceptive potentials of dorsal horn units, these appearing much later (7 seconds), and the complete absence of after-sensation at the end of stimulation. This experiment was reproduced many times by both groups of scientists, comparable results having been obtained every time.

From the very beginning, it was clear in all interventions under acupuncture analgesia on man and animals that acupuncture analgesia is not effective at once, but rather, has a latency phase, this requiring 5-10 minutes when manual stimulation is used, and 20-40 minutes when electrical stimulation is used. Therefore, the mode of action cannot possibly be of a purely neural nature, but rather, transmitter substances must also be called into action.

Manipulation of Neurotransmitters by Acupuncture

Not too long ago, studies by *Riederer, Tenk, Werner, Birkmayer, Bischko, Rett,* and *Krisper* were published on the manipulation of neurotransmitters via acupuncture. I find these of especial importance, as they alone seem to have presented the first plausible explanation for the long-term effects of acupuncture therapy. In anesthesiology, we find an uninterrupted stimulus chain being an absolute prerequisite for the achievement of the analgesic effect. This clearly implies the action of a predominately neural mechanism.

Acupuncture as therapy must be strictly distinguished from acupuncture analgesia both in regard to the technique and to the theoretical foundations thereof; its relatively long-term effects can with certainty not be explained by predominately neural mechanisms. Of much greater importance in regard to acupunctural therapy seems to be the fact that treatment of points which are noteworthy mainly by virtue of the receptor structures they contain results in a greater release of serotonin than does treatment of points having predominately effector structures.

These data shed new light on the aforementioned studies done by *Kellner,* and contribute to better comprehension of the point combinations presented herein.

Similar investigations were carried out by *Krötlinger* in regard to other biochemical parameters (phosphates, 17-ketosteroids, potassium), all of which produced the same or similar results, with the sole exception of calcium. For details, see „Handbuch der Akupunktur und Aurikulotherapie" (Karl F. Haug Publishers).

Recently, studies by *Snyder, Pomeranz* et al. have been published on opiate receptors, especially in the periaqueductal gray matter, and also in other parts of the brain, spinal cord, and indeed, other organs. The taking of opiates not being a part of common daily life, attention was focused on the investigation of morphine-like substances produced within the body, called endorphin and encephalin. These serve stress response and are released by acupuncture to a high degree. Morphine antidotes, such as naloxone, can inhibit the effect of parenteral doses of morphine, as well as of an efficacious acupuncture analgesia, but not of hypnosis, the oscillogram of which in the EEG differs from that under acupuncture analgesia *(Saletu)*. If nothing else does, this definitely refutes the views expounded on the subject by *Dotzauer* and *Prokop*.

A study by *Gilly, Herkner, Pauser,* and *Steinbereithner* based on the aforementioned experiments on cats revealed practically the same results being achieved in regard to the nociceptive potentials via acupuncture as via parenteral administration of β-endorphin. We may therefore assume that acupuncture can activate neurophysiologic and biochemical parameters.

We purported the effect of biochemical factors from the very beginning, this for three reasons:

1. the effect's prolonged latency period,
2. the relative stability of vital parameters, these rendering acupuncture analgesia of particular interest for anesthesia of problem cases (there is, as a rule, only a slight increase in blood pressure, up to 20 mm/Hg, in the initial phase),
3. the – actually incomprehensible – indifference, indeed at times even somnolent behavior of the – completely conscious – patient during surgery.

Especially the latter aspect, as well as the reported sensations of warmth and heaviness proceeding from the inserted acupuncture needles, may have initially led some critics of the method to the erroneous conclusion that acupuncture is a type of induced hypnosis, the latter evoking similar symptoms.

Already a long time ago, attempts were made to find a way of sparing the patient the – hardly perceptible – pain caused by needling. *Voll* tried with the electro-acupuncture method bearing his name. Already in the late 50's, *Feucht* experimented with foil made of different metals, these adhering to skin zones and points with an adhesive underlayer. Ultrasound and vibratory devices were used, producing unsatisfactory results. Finally, the laser beam came into use, however, not that used for surgery, but rather, that used in communications technology, having an output of 2 mW. We tested instruments from various manufacturers for many years. The results: absolute efficacy in therapy, but ineffectiveness in the treatment of paralyses and for acupuncture analgesia. Laser treatment is completely painless, and therefore, particularly suited for treatment of children and hypersensitive patients, as well as for macerating dermatologic disorders. Laser therapy is completely risk-free for both patient and physician. It was once again the histologist, *Kellner*, who carried out the fundamental investigations thereupon. On the skin of pigs, he demonstrated that even during constant laser stimulation from a distance of 20 cm for hours at a time, an approx. 0.3 mm depth of penetration was reached after 5 seconds, a depth of approx. 0.7 mm after 10 seconds, and after 15 seconds, a depth of only approx. 0.4 mm could be maintained. Even hours later, no tissular injury could be determined, of the eye included, it having been irradiated with the punctiform laser beam for four hours. When the pen of the instrument is applied directly to the skin, the depth of penetration is about 1 mm, the length of application per point being 15-20 seconds. The same acupuncture points are used as in needling.

The development of laser acupuncture brought with it new aspects, especially in regard to the use of acupuncture in pediatrics. An example is the results obtained by *Liertzer* in the treatment of juvenile asthma, which could be spirometrically verified.

In a unique experiment based on data from *Akabane* and *Voll*, *Krötlinger* demonstrated that the electric potential of all points of a meridian is changed upon stimulation of a point belonging to that meridian, be it via needling or laser beam; nevertheless, the potential even of neighboring points of another meridian remains unchanged. The meridians have already been discussed herein.

Due to the fact that two meridians traverse, for example, the thumb, corresponding to the same segment in the spinal column, one can no longer rightly speak today of a sole segmental dependency of acupuncture, as my former pupil, *Wancura*, assumed, without, however, having presented corresponding experimental data.

I stated earlier that therapeutic acupuncture is a, or better said, **the** regulative therapy. This assumption as well can be substantiated by a number of examples and experiments.

Already quite some time ago, *Kubista* and *Kucera* demonstrated that acupuncture, administered to primiparae prior to delivery, was able to reduce the duration of labour by 50% in comparison to a control group. These results were tocographically verified by *Zerobin* and *Kothbauer* in animal experiments on cows by means of sensors implanted in the uterus. Comparative trials revealed that cows treated with acupuncture demonstrated labor contractions strictly from fundus to cervix only, whereas the untreated animals also had contractions of a circular nature, and even from cervix to fundus, this, of course, prolonging delivery.

There have also been a number of investigations on a typical phenomenon in acupuncture briefly mentioned heretofore, the stabilization of vital parameters. This is another reason for acupuncture analgesia's being mainly used today in cardiac surgery and problem cases. Therewith, the general condition of such patients is incomparably better; their breathing, bowel, and urinary actions are not irritated, even following abdominal surgery. In connection therewith, I would like to cite *Chiang,* who studied 2 groups of 9 cats each, one of which was acupunctured on the shock point (on the philtrum), and the other not. All of the animals were put into hemorrhagic shock, and the withdrawn blood reinfused immediately thereafter over a period of one hour. None of the untreated animals survived the procedure. Of those treated with acupuncture, only one died after four hours.

I shall not go into pharma-acupuncture here. We know that acupuncture enhances the effect of simultaneously administered drugs. Use thereof is made by injecting i.c. or s.c. subdoses of indicated substances into acupuncture points.

Upon insertion of the needle, red halos appear on the skin around it, the skin temperature increasing 1-2°C. These halos were considered to be a histamine effect. However, they even appeared to nearly the same degree of intensity under parenteral and local administration of high doses of antihistamines *(Bischko, Stöckl).* Likewise, i.v. blood tests prior to acupuncture and every 5 minutes thereafter (for one hour) revealed no significant changes *(Skorczyk).* What, then, caused the temperature increase? *Kellner* had already postulated in 1965 that acupuncture produces a change in arterio-venous anastomosis. Both he himself, as well as the Soviet school *(Durinjan),* were able to verify his assumption by means of thermography. The latter demonstrated that individual acupuncture points call forth selective effects appropriate to the respective organ or disease. This shed new light on the cited sensation of warmth.

However, that is not necessarily the final word on the subject. *Popp* reported on information transmission in biological systems and the extremely weak photon emission thereof. He and his coworker, *Ruth,* expand the original experiment done by the Russian scientist, *Gurwitsch.* The latter placed the roots of onion sprouts very close together and observed that these mutally supported each other in growth. When separated by a pane of glass, this process did not take place. It did, however, when the pane was of quartz. *Gurwitsch* inferred therefrom that ultraviolet rays must be a decisive factor, these, as we know, not penetrating glass. The extremely weak photon emission, however, is 10^{40} times stronger than heat rays and therefore seems – with feedback effect of course – capable of regulating biochemical processes in the cells. The conclusion may be drawn that coded response systems must be present in biochemical regulatory processes.

With this future-oriented contribution, which is of particular significance for laser therapy, I would like to close the chapter on scientific data on acupuncture, being fully aware of not having listed everything on the subject, nor gone into much detail.

I have presented these data for the sole purpose of substantiating my initial "yes" to the question of whether acupuncture has a justified place in our, modern times, and to show you, the reader, that the method you have elected to study is neither mystic, occult, nor disreputable.

REFERENCES

Abele, U.: Paper presented at the yearly meeting of the "Deutsche Gesellschaft für Akupuntur", 1968.

Akabane, N.: Cited by *Bachmann* in: Leitfaden der Akupunktur. Karl F. Haug Publishers. Ulm/Donau 1961.

Aschner, B.: Lehrbuch der Konstitutionskrankheiten. Hippokrates. Stuttgart 1953.

Bachmann, G.: Leitfaden der Akupunktur. Karl F. Haug Publishers. Ulm/Donau 1961.

Baunscheidt, C.: Der Baunscheidtismus. Bonn 1860.

Bergsmann, O.: Objektivierung der Akupunktur als Problem der Regulationsphysiologie. Karl F. Haug Publishers. Heidelberg 1974.

Bischko, J.: Einführung in die Akupunktur. 13th ed. Karl F. Haug Publishers. Heidelberg 1983.

Bischko, J.: An Introduction to Acupuncture. 1st ed. Karl F. Haug Publishers. Heidelberg 1978.

Bischko, J.: Akupunktur für Fortgeschrittene. 7th ed. Karl F. Haug Publishers. Heidelberg 1981.

Bischko, J., Meng, A.: Akupunktur für mäßig Fortgeschrittene. 4th ed. Karl F. Haug Publishers. Heidelberg 1985.

Bischko, J., Meng, A.: Intermediate Acupuncture (in preparation). Karl F. Haug Publishers. Heidelberg.

Bischko, J., Stöckl, W.: Unpublished data.

Bong Han, K.: On the Kyungrak System. Foreign Languages Publishing House. Kyungrak System and Theory of Sanal. Medical Science Press. Pyöngyang. Korea, DPRK 1964.

Bratu, I., Stoicescu, C., Prodescu, V.: Der Wert der Ermittlung des elektrischen Widerstands des Hautgewebes bei der Akupunktur. Deutsche Zeitschrift für Akupunktur 6 (1960) 125.

Busse, U., Busse, P.: Akupunkturfibel, Die Praxis der chinesischen Akupunkturlehre. Pflaum. Munich 1975.

Chamfrault, A. and M.: Traité de médecine chinoise. Editions Coquemard 1954.

Chiang (Phys. Institute, Shanghai): pers. communication.

De la Fuye, F.: Traité d'Acupuncture. Librairie Le François. Paris 1956.

De Tymowski, J.M.: Le Massage chinois. 1960.

Dickhaus, H., Pauser, G., Zimmermann, M.: Hemmung im Rückenmark, ein neurophysiologischer Wirkungsmechanismus bei der Hypalgesie durch Stimulationsakupunktur. Wiener klinische Wochenschrift 90, 2 (1978) 59.

Dotzauer, G., Prokop, O.: Die Akupunktur. Gustav Fischer. Stuttgart 1979.

Durinjan, R.A.: Pers. communication.

Feucht, G.: Beeinflussung lokaler Regulationsstörungen mit Edelmetallfolien. Erfahrungsheilkunde 9 (1972) 281.

Fleischhacker, H.: Klinik der Herderkrankungen. Therapiewoche 15, 24 (1965) 1274.

Foerster, O.: Resection of the posterior spinal nervous roots in the treatment of gastric and spastic paralysis. Proc. roy. Soc. Med. 4 (1911) 226.

Fujita, R., Minami, S.: Experimentelle Untersuchungen über die Wirkung von Gold- und Silbernadeln besonders hinsichtlich tonifizierender und sedierender Wirkung. Deutsche Zeitschrift für Akupunktur 9-10 (1959) 97.

Gilly, H.: Rechnerunterstützte Datenauswertung von neurophysiologischen Experimenten zur Quantifizierung der Analgesiewirkung nach Modellakupunktur. Deutsche Zeitschrift für Akupunktur 22 (1976) 69.

Gleditsch, J.M.: Die Mundakupunktur. WBV Biologisch-Medizinische Verlagsgesellschaft. Schorndrof 1979.

Gross, D.: Die Nase als nervaler Rezeptor. Medizinische Klinik 42 (1953) 1549.

Gurwitsch, A.: Cited by *Popp:* Krank sein – wenn Zellen nicht mehr miteinander reden. Bild der Wissenschaft 8 (1977) 90.

Hoff, F.: Steuerungseinrichtungen des Organismus in Gesundheit und Krankheit. G. Thieme. Stuttgart, New York 1943.

Hoff, F.: Klinische Physiologie und Pathologie. G. Thieme. Stuttgart, New York 1957.

Hoff, F.: Pers. communication.

Keidel, W.D.: Elektronarkose und Akupunktur aus der Sicht der Neurophysiologie. Klinikarzt 4 (1975) 277.

Kellner, G.: Bau und Funktion der Haut. Deutsche Zeitschrift für Akupunktur 1 (1966) 1.

Kellner, G.: Cited by *Bischko:* Use of the Laser Beam in Acupuncture. Acupuncture & Electro-Therapeut. Res., Int. J., Vol. 5 (1980) 29.

Klauser, G.: Verschiedene Aspekte der Raucherentwöhnung durch Akupunktur. Deutsche Zeitschrift für Akupunktur 4 (1980) 78.

Kokoschinegg, P.: Biophysik in der Akupunktur. Deutsche Zeitschrift für Akupunktur 3 (1980) 60.

Kokoschinegg, P.: Grundlagen der Laserbehandlung und der bioelektrischen Meßtechnik. Erfahrungsheilkunde 7 (1979) 521.

Konnen, N.: Pers. communication.

Kothbauer, O.: Akupunktur und Neuraltherapie zur Sterilitätsbehandlung des Rindes. Karl F. Haug Publishers. Heidelberg 1978.

Kothbauer, O.: Film Discussion of the Operation on the Udder Teats of the Cow under Acupuncture Analgesia. Proceedings of the Second French, Italian, and Austrian Congress, Acupuncture and Auricular Therapy. Vienna, June 13-15, 1975 (Ed.: *J. Bischko).*

H. Egermann. Vienna, p. 63.

Kothbauer, O., Zerobin, K.: Die Verifizierung des Akupunkturreizes mittels tokographischer Untersuchungen auf dem Uterus des Rindes während der Geburts- und Puerperalphase. Deutsche Zeitschrift für Akupunktur 4 (1977) 111.

Kropej, H.: The Fundamentals of Ear Acupuncture. 2nd ed. Karl F. Haug Publishers. Heidelberg 1984.

Krötlinger, M.: Neuere Meßergebnisse zum Vorhandensein der Meridiane. Deutsche Zeitschrift für Akupunktur 3 (1978) 75.

Krötlinger, M.: On the Use of the Laser in Acupuncture. Acupuncture & Electro-Therapeutics Res., Int. J., Vol. 5 (1980) 297.

Krötlinger, M.: Pharmaakupunktur bei Gelenksbeschwerden in der Allgemeinpraxis. Deutsche Zeitschrift für Akupunktur 1 (1978) 14.

Krötlinger, M.: Vorläufige Mitteilung zur theoretischen Erklärung der Akupunkturwirkung. Deutsche Zeitschrift für Akupunktur 6 (1978) 151.

Kubista, E., Kucera, H.: Acupuncture as a Method of Preparation in Obstetrics. Am. J. Chin. Med. 2, 3 (1974) 283.

Lang, W.: Über das Wesen der Meridiane in neurologischer Sicht. Deutsche Zeitschrift für Akupunktur 3 (1968) 65.

Liertzer, H.: Laserakupunktur in der Kinderheilkunde am Beispiel des Asthma bronchiale. Deutsche Zeitschrift für Akupunktur 2 (1980) 36.

Lutz, F., Pischinger, A.: Wiener Medizinische Wochenschrift **99** (1949) 437.

Majer, E.H.: Zur Gefäßversorgung der oberen Luftwege, Otologia Fukuoko **13,** 2 (1967) 92.

Majer, E.H., Bischko, J.: Zur Akupunktur bei Tonsillenoperationen. Arch. klin. exp. Ohr.-, Nas.- u. Kehlk.-Heilk. 205 (1973) 280.

Mann, F.: The Ancient Chinese Art of Healing. Heinemann Medical. London 1962.

Mann, F.: The Treatment of Disease by Acupuncture. Heinemann Medical. London 1963.

Maresch, O.: Das elektrische Verhalten der Haut. Deutsche Zeitschrift für Akupuntur, 2 (1966) 38.

Meng, A.: Die traditionelle chinesische Massage. 2nd ed. Karl F. Haug Publishers. Heidelberg 1984.

Nakatani, Y.: Über den Wirkungsunterschied zwischen der Gold- und Silbernadel bei der Akupunktur. Deutsche Zeitschrift für Akupunktur 1 (1960) 16.

Nogier, P.F.M.: Traité d'Auriculothérapie. Ed. Maisonneuve. Sainte Ruffine 1969.

Pauser, G.: Neurophysiologische und neuropharmakologische Untersuchungen über (mögliche) Mechanismen der peripheren Stimulationsanalgesie. Wiener klinische Wochenschrift 92, Supplement 113 (1980) 3.

Pauser, G. Reichman, Ch., Baum, M., Benzer, H., Haider, W., Thoma, H.: Beeinflussung der Schmerzempfindung des Schmerzgefühls und der vegetativen Lage des Organismus unter Akupunkturanalgesie. Wiener klinische Wochenschrift 87 (1975) 25.

Petricek, E., Zeitler, H.: Neue Systematische Ordnung der Neu-Punkte. Karl F. Haug Publishers. Heidelberg 1976.

Pischinger, A.: Das System der Grundregulation. 4th. ed. Karl F. Haug Publishers. Heidelberg 1983.

Pomeranz, B.: Akupunkturwirkung durch Ausschüttung von Enzephalinen und Endorphinen im Gehirn. New Scientist 73 (1977) 12; cited by *D. Marthaler.*

Popp, F.A.: Krank sein – wenn Zellen nicht mehr miteinander reden. Bild der Wissenschaft 8 (1977) 90.

Popp, F.A., Strauss, V.E.: So könnte Krebs entstehen. Biophysikalische Zellforschung – Hoffnung für Millionen? Deutsche Verlags-Anstalt. Stuttgart 1977.

Prinzing, G.: Über die unterschiedliche Wirkung der Gold- und Silbernadel in der Akupunktur. Deutsche Zeitschrift für Akupunktur 2 (1960) 29.

Puder, N.: Cited by *Bergsmann.*

Quaglia-Senta, A.: L'Acupuncture chinoise. Maisonneuve. Paris 1969.

Riederer, P., Tenk, H., Werner, H., Bischko, J., Rett, A., Krsiper, H.: Manipulation of Neurotransmitters by Acupuncture. J. of Neural Transmission 37 (1975) 81.

Saletu, B., Brown, M., Stern, J., Sletten, I., Ulett, G.: Hypno-Analgesia and Acupuncture Analgesia: A Neurophysiological Reality? Neuropsychobiology 1 (1975) 218.

Schmidt, H.: Akupunkturtherapie nach der chinesischen Typenlehre. Hippokrates, Stuttgart 1978.

Schroeder, J.: Erfahrungsbericht. Deutsche Zeitschrift für Akupunktur 11-12 (1957) 133.

Selye, N.: Cited by *Bischko* in Akupunktur und Stress. Deutsche Zeitschrift für Akupunktur 11-12 (1955) 124.

Skorczyk, W.: Pers. communication.

Snyder, O.: Cited in "Euromed" – das europäisch-medizinische Magazin 21 (1976).

Soulié de Morant, G.: La vera agopuntura cinese. Bocca. Milan 1943.

Stacher, A.: Therapiewoche **15,** 24 (1965) 1278.

Stacher, A.: Pers. communication.

Szillard, N.: Pers. communication.

Te Suck Song: Über die verschiedene Wirkung der Gold- und Silbernadel. Deutsche Zeitschrift für Akupunktur 7-8 (1959) 84.

Voll, A.: Topographische Lage der Meßpunkte der Elektro-Akupunktur. Medizinisch-Literarische Verlagsgesellschaft. Uelzen 1976.

Wehlend, N.: Paper presented at the Second World Congress on Acupuncture. Paris 1969.

Wogralik, W.G.: Die klinisch physiologischen Grundlagen der Nadelungstherapie und der Moxa bei inneren Erkrankungen, Deutsche Zeitschrift für Akupunktur 5 (1960) 97.

Yanagiya, S.: Familiengeheime Ein-Stich-Akupunktur. 6th ed. Karl F. Haug Publishers. Heidelberg 1981.

Zeitler, H.: Einführung in die Schädelakupunktur. 2nd ed. Karl F. Haug Publishers. Heidelberg 1978.

Zottermann, Y.: Touch, pain and tickling, an electrophysiological investigation on cutaneous sensory nerves. J. Physiol. (1939) 95.

All standard acupuncture textbooks were consulted in regard to their fundamental statements, in particular:

Stiefvater, E.W.: Praxis der Akupunktur, 5th revised ed. of Akupunktur als Neuraltherapie. Karl F. Haug Publishers. Heidelberg 1974.

Stiefvater, E.W. and *I.:* Acupuncture charts, 7th ed. Karl F. Haug Publishers. Heidelberg 1982.

Stiefvater, E.W.: Was ist Akupunktur? 2nd ed. Karl F. Haug Publishers. Heidelberg 1973.

Ten Rhyne, W.: Die Akupunktur des Ten Rhyne. Reissued with comments by Dr. *Erich W. Stiefvater.* Karl F. Haug Publishers. Ulm/Donau 1955.

Due to the recent rapid development of acupuncture we would like to particularly recommend the "Handbuch für Akupunktur und Auriculotherapie," Karl F. Haug Publishers, ring-book and single editions, particularly the works by *Kropej, Krötlinger, Meng, Petricek,* and *Zeitler.*

We also refer you to the "Deutsche Zeitschrift für Akupunktur" (Ed.: *J. Bischko),* which, of course being a journal, is able to publish new studies or research faster than a book (Karl F. Haug Publishers, Heidelberg).

And finally, another note. The number of books and publications (in German-speaking countries as well) which are either based on "even older" or "even newer" Chinese works is growing constantly.

These works are certainly of great interest because of China's special position in regard to acupuncture in the past as well as now in the People's Republic. However, the differences between China and the Western world must be kept in mind (medical jurisprudence, different bodily structure, other social conditions, etc.).

Therefore, our endeavor to create a European, or better, Western, form of acupuncture seems to us to be justified.

Superficial needle insertion, which we recommend (in constrast to original Chinese data) is even considered correct in China today. The original guideline was: Superficial needle insertion for persons with chronic illnesses, for persons who do not perform hard physical work, for those who suffer from nervous tension, and for children or old persons. More than 90% of our patients in the West fit those descriptions.

Appendix

OVERVIEW OF THE MERIDIANS BY H. LIERTZER

Meridian	H	SI	B	K	P	3H	G	Li	Lu	LI	St	SP
Tonification Point	H9	SI3	B67	K7	P9	3H3	G43	Li8	Lu9	LI11	St41	SP2
Sedation Point	H7	SI8	B65	K1,2	P7	3H10	G38	Li2	Lu5	LI2,3	St45	SP5
Source Point	H7	SI4	B64	K3	P7	3H4	G40	Li3	Lu9	LI4	St42	SP3
Passage Point	H5	SI7	B58	K4	P6	3H5	G37	Li6	Lu7	LI6	St40	SP4
Concurring Point	B15	B27	B28	B23	B14	B22	B19	B18	B13	B24	B21	B20
Alarm Point	CV14	CV4	CV3	G25	P1 K11	CV5 CV7 CV12 CV17	G23 G24	Li14	Lu1	St25	CV12	SP15 Li13
Maximum Time	noon-2pm	2-4pm	4-6pm	6-8pm	8-10pm	10pm-midnight	midnight-2am	2-4am	4-6am	6-8am	8-10am	10am-noon

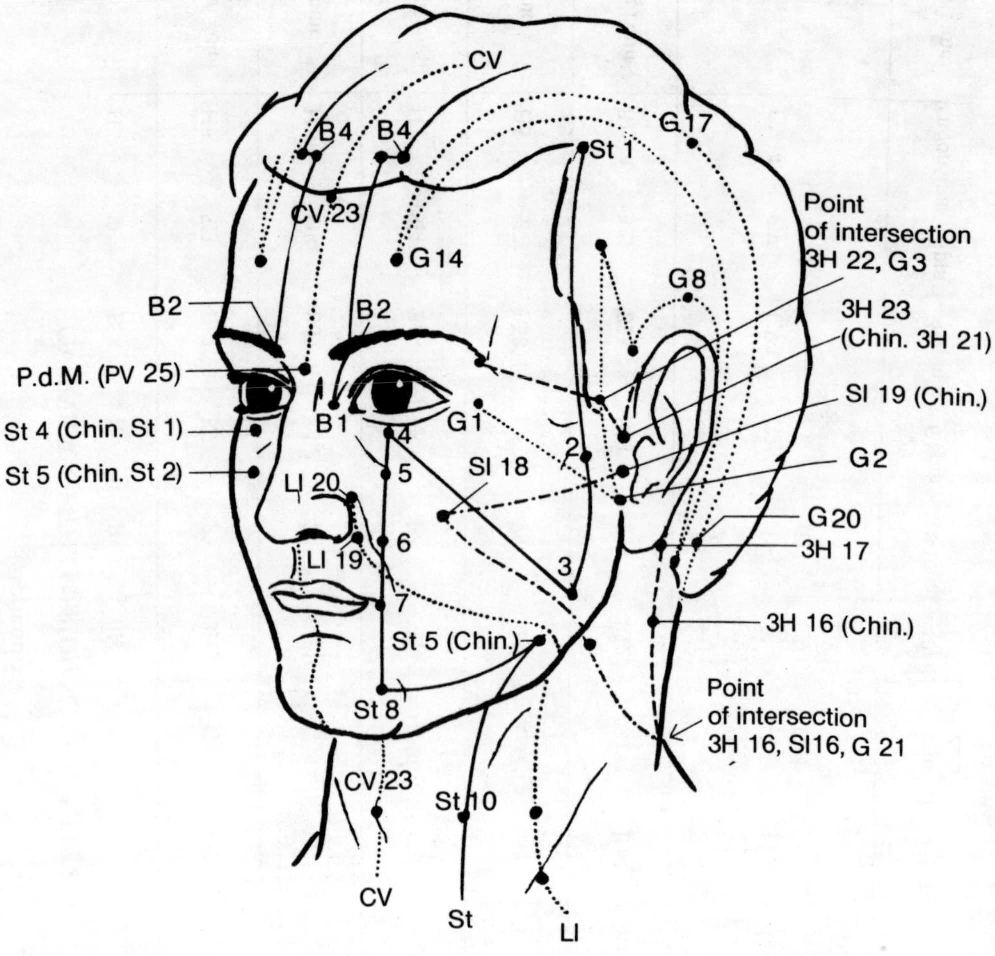
CV
B4
B4
G17
St 1
CV 23
Point
of intersection
3H 22, G3
G14
G8
B2
B2
3H 23
(Chin. 3H 21)
P.d.M. (PV 25)
SI 19 (Chin.)
St 4 (Chin. St 1)
B1
G1
4
2
G2
St 5 (Chin. St 2)
5
SI 18
LI 20
G20
6
3H 17
LI 19
3
7
3H 16 (Chin.)
St 5 (Chin.)
Point
of intersection
3H 16, SI16, G 21
St 8
CV 23
St 10
CV
St
LI

Fig. 19

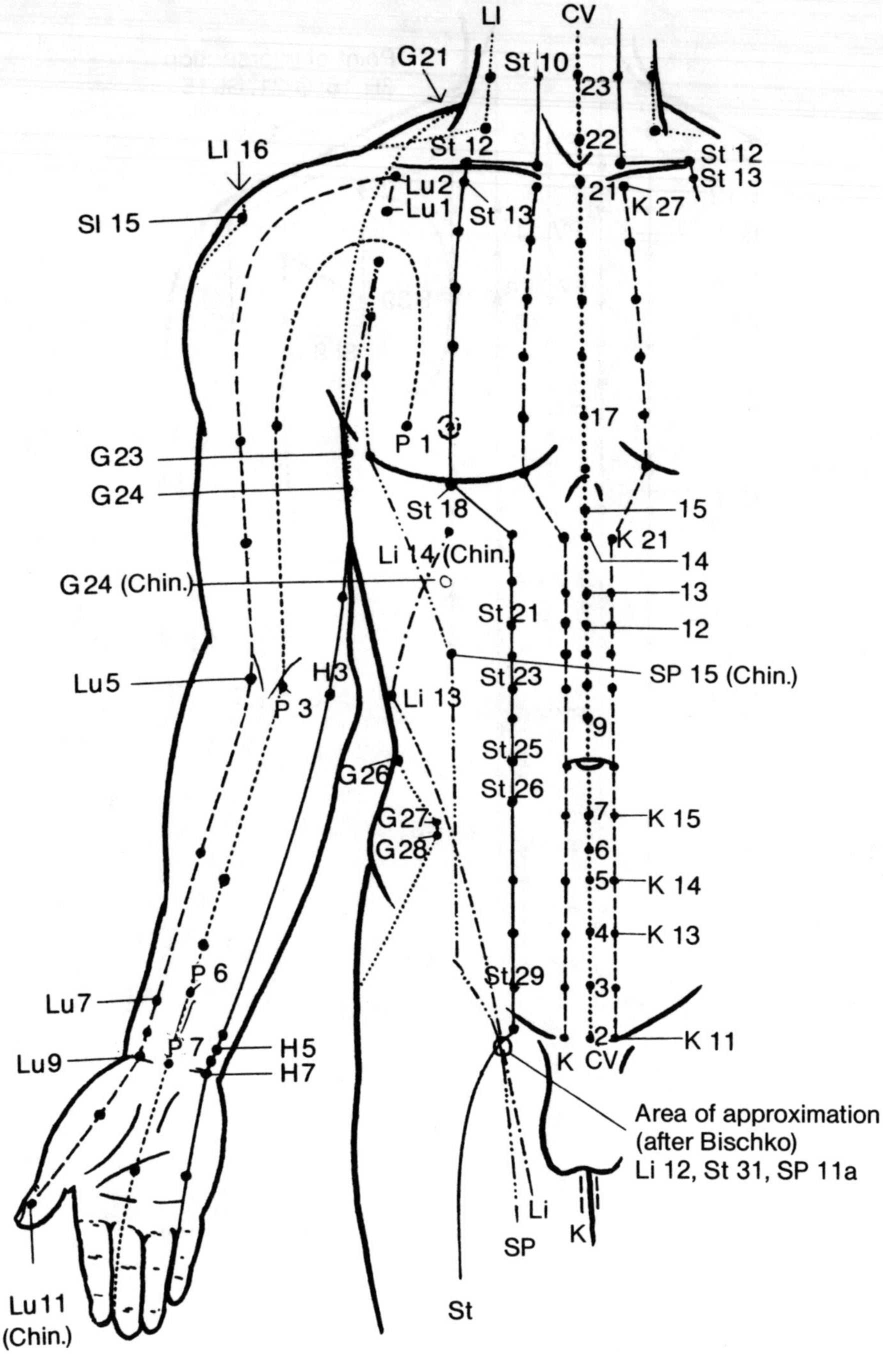

LI
CV
G21
St 10
23
22
21
LI 16
St 12
St 12
St 13
Lu2
Lu1
St 13
K 27
SI 15
17
P 1
G23
G24
St 18
15
K 21
14
Li 14 (Chin.)
G24 (Chin.)
13
St 21
12
SP 15 (Chin.)
Lu5
H3
St 23
P 3
Li 13
9
St 25
G26
St 26
G27
7
K 15
G28
6
5
K 14
4
K 13
P 6
St 29
3
Lu7
2
K 11
P 7
H5
Lu9
H7
K
CV
Area of approximation
(after Bischko)
Li 12, St 31, SP 11a
Li
SP
K
St
Lu11
(Chin.)

Fig. 20

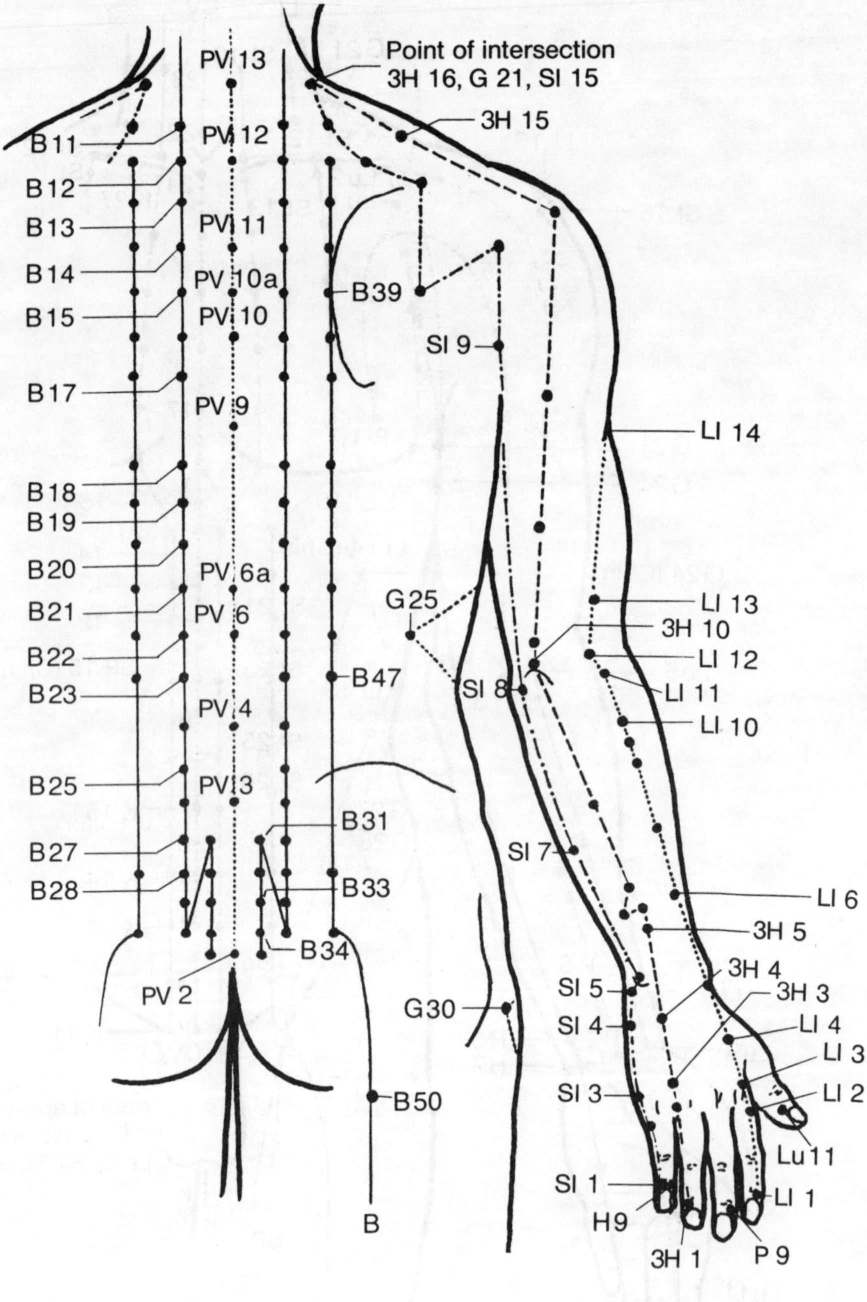

Point of intersection
3H 16, G 21, SI 15
3H 15
PV 13
PV 12
PV 11
PV 10a
PV 10
PV 9
PV 6a
PV 6
PV 4
PV 3
PV 2
B 11
B 12
B 13
B 14
B 15
B 17
B 18
B 19
B 20
B 21
B 22
B 23
B 25
B 27
B 28
B 31
B 33
B 34
B 39
B 47
B 50
B
SI 9
LI 14
G 25
LI 13
3H 10
LI 12
SI 8
LI 11
LI 10
SI 7
LI 6
3H 5
3H 4
3H 3
SI 5
SI 4
LI 4
LI 3
G 30
SI 3
LI 2
Lu 11
SI 1
LI 1
H 9
3H 1
P 9

Fig. 21

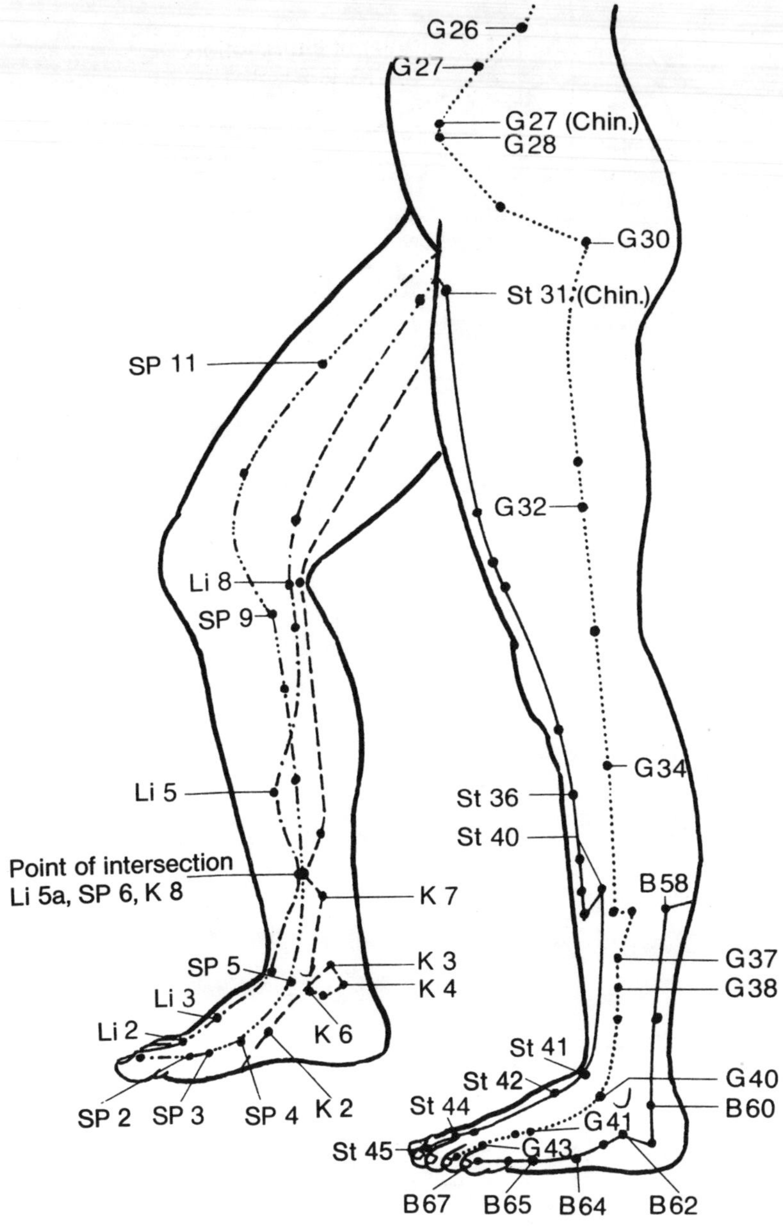
G 26
G 27
G 27 (Chin.)
G 28
G 30
St 31 (Chin.)
SP 11
G 32
Li 8
SP 9
G 34
Li 5
St 36
St 40
Point of intersection
Li 5a, SP 6, K 8
K 7
B 58
SP 5
K 3
G 37
Li 3
K 4
G 38
Li 2
K 6
St 41
St 42
G 40
SP 2
SP 3
SP 4
K 2
St 44
B 60
G 41
St 45
G 43
B 67
B 65
B 64
B 62

Fig. 22